STAY HEALTHY, LIVE LONGER, SPEND WISELY

Making Intelligent Choices in America's Healthcare System

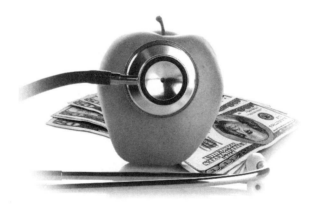

Davis Liu, M.D.

Stetho Publishing
Sacramento, CA

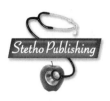

Published by:
Stetho Publishing
PO Box 254450
Sacramento, CA 95865-4450

Stay Healthy, Live Longer, Spend Wisely:
Making Intelligent Choices in America's Healthcare System

By Davis Liu, M.D.

Copyright © 2008 by Davis Liu, M.D.

Publisher's Cataloging-In-Publication Data
(Prepared by The Donohue Group, Inc.)

Liu, Davis.
  Stay healthy, live longer, spend wisely : making intelligent choices in America's healthcare system / Davis Liu.

  p. ; cm.

  Includes bibliographical references and index.
  ISBN-13: 978-0-9793512-0-4
  ISBN-10: 0-9793512-0-0

  1. Patient education—United States—Handbooks, manuals, etc. 2. Medical care— United States—Handbooks, manuals, etc. 3. Consumer education—United States— Handbooks, manuals, etc. 4. Health insurance—United States— Handbooks, manuals, etc. 5. Physician and patient—United States—Handbooks, manuals, etc. I. Title.

R727.4 .L58 2008
615.5/07/1   2007903308

Book and cover design by Peri Poloni-Gabriel, Knockout Design, www.knockoutbooks.com
Index by Clive Pyne Book Indexing Services.
Edited by Gail M. Kearns, To Press and Beyond, www.topressandbeyond.com
Book production coordinated by To Press and Beyond

Printed in the United States of America

Contents

PART FOUR: Meet Your Medical Team — 135

ACKNOWLEDGEMENTS

I would like to thank Paul Erlich, M.D, Oli Mittermaier, John Martin, Ahmet Ucmakli, M.D, and Robert M. Wachter, M.D. for their advice on book writing.

I appreciate the help from Francis Mataac, Kathleen Liu, and Sharon Levine, M.D. for their input on the manuscript, as well as the important peer reviews by Dr. Erlich and Ernie Bodai, M.D., both respected and busy practicing clinicians who work diligently outside the office increasing public awareness on asthma and breast cancer awareness and research respectively. This book could not have been produced without the skills, editing, and coordination provided by Gail M. Kearns at To Press and Beyond (www.topressandbeyond.com).

I am fortunate to be a practicing primary care physician at the Permanente Medical Group, which is led by an extraordinary and inspirational leader, Robert Pearl, M.D. Dr. Pearl made me realize that high quality accessible and affordable health care is not consistently delivered in our country and our medical group must continue to be a leader to initiate change so that everyone has an equal opportunity to get the best care our American healthcare system has to offer.

I am tremendously grateful to my parents, who had the courage to emigrate from Taiwan and start a new life first in Canada and then the United States, and begin a family. Despite being isolated from family and friends and immersed in a foreign culture and language, they had the foresight to know that their enormous sacrifice, as well as many which followed, would provide my siblings and me opportunities that would exceed anything we could ever imagine.

I appreciate my three siblings, Karen, Kathleen, and Dennis, who continue to keep me grounded and naturally influenced the way I am today. Understandably, they periodically call for medical advice, but still don't seem to take me seriously.

Life would not be as enjoyable without my daughter, Emma, who was born during the time I was working on this book. Through her eyes, she reminds me of the wonder and joy it is to be a child and the potential of what life has to offer.

Finally, I am especially thankful to my wife, Jocelyn, who throughout this multi-year process, which at times seemed like it would never end, remained supportive. I can't imagine going through this journey we call life with anyone else.

THE DOCTOR IS IN

The U.S. healthcare system is in crisis. As it currently exists, it will risk people's financial wellbeing and their ability to pay for care, which will ultimately impact their physical health.

Although our healthcare system remains the world's most expensive, it provides medical care that lags behind that of many nations and is increasingly unaffordable to millions of Americans. Annually, tens of thousands of patients die prematurely, not due to medical errors, but because basic and well-known preventive interventions are not practiced consistently across the country. Our fragmented system adds cost and wastes time with the duplication of tests and procedures.

Physicians do not have enough time to educate their patients about everything they need to do to stay healthy. The public is confronted with a bewildering number of pharmaceutical products, insurance plans, and alternative therapies, and often is confused about what to do. Employers are asking their employees to pay more for less coverage or are dropping their benefits completely. Although there are organizations trying to improve the quality of the healthcare system, it is still far from being fixed. Our government has no long-term strategy for overhauling the system.

From personal and professional experience, I see how the complexity of the system scares and intimidates individuals. Patients want to do the right thing but they are overwhelmed with too many choices and concerned about escalating costs, so they avoid a system that is not user friendly. Being a physician, I know how to get the most out of our healthcare system, find the right care, and avoid unnecessary costs. I often advise family, friends, and patients based on these insights.

While I don't know how to fix our healthcare crisis, I want to share my knowledge with you to help provide you and your family the best chance of getting the most out of our healthcare system. Until our healthcare system undergoes major reforms, it will favor those with adequate funds and the know-how on getting the right care. Educate yourself so that you will make the right choices and thus protect your physical health and financial future.

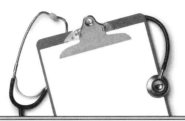

DISCLAIMER

This book provides general medical, health insurance, and financial information that are meant to inform and educate the reader. Readers should consult with their doctors, human resources staff, insurance brokers, accountants, and financial advisors about their specific situations, as this book does not replace their counsel.

It is sold with the understanding that the publisher and author shall neither have the liability nor responsibility to anyone who feels that information in this book caused, directly or indirectly, any loss or damage.

The opinions and views are those of the author and do not reflect those of the Permanente Medical Group. The author has made every attempt to eliminate typos and misspellings.

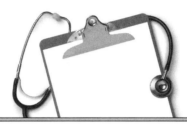

A NOTE TO THE READER

You may notice, as a matter of convention, I will refer to doctors using the pronoun he or him. This is for convenience. Certainly there are many more female physicians today, and my medical school over the past few years has had more female medical students than male.

INTRODUCTION

Despite paying more for health insurance, you are getting less. Every year, a bewildering number of choices in insurance plans, health-care providers, medications, and treatment options, all touted as being the best, confront you. Yet unlike other items you purchase, there is not an easy way for you to compare whether you are getting the right insurance plan, treatment, medication or even if you're seeing the right kind of doctor.

Unfortunately, the future looks even bleaker. From 2000 to 2005, health insurance premiums have increased 73 percent as compared to inflation (14 percent) and wage increases (15 percent), and they are expected to continue to rise.[1] Although as a nation we spend more on health care per capita than any other country in the world, we cannot claim that we live the longest. The government doesn't seem interested in truly reforming the healthcare system. Sadly, this indifference is splitting our nation into two groups — the haves and the have-nots. Those who have enough money to pay for more comprehensive health insurance or those who have the knowledge on how to spend their money wisely will have the advantage. Those with inadequate money or knowledge could find that their health suffers. Consider the current problems:

➤ In 2005, one in five Americans (21 percent) reported having an overdue medical bill. Almost three out of ten (29 percent) skipped medical tests, cut medications, or skipped doses due to cost. A majority (56 percent) felt their medical condition worsened as a result. Eighteen percent said healthcare costs were the largest expense outside of rent or mortgage.[2]

➤ In 2005, it was estimated that annually 83,000 Americans died prematurely, not because of hospital errors, misdiagnoses, or negligence but because they did not get care in accordance with guidelines from national expert committees, and they did not get the care backed by scientific evidence and research. Had they enrolled in a high performing health care plan, it is very likely these deaths could have been avoided.[3]

➤ A 2003 report noted that 80 percent of employers felt that the *cost* of a health plan was a very important factor, while only 3 percent felt that health care *quality* was as important.

➤ The Employee Benefit Research Institute predicts that a couple retiring in 2006 will need $295,000 to fund health insurance premiums and out-of-pocket expenses.[4] For future retirees, the picture is bleak with predictions that health care costs will eat up 20 percent of pre-retirement income.

➤ Cutting your health costs indiscriminately can hurt your health: a June 2004 report showed that patients with chronic preexisting medical conditions who curtailed their prescription medications because of cost were 76 percent more likely to suffer a significant decline in their overall health, and 50 percent more likely to have a nonfatal heart attack or stroke than those who did not cut back.

Your instincts are right. You are getting less for more. You spend weeks waiting for an appointment. The office co-pays are going up and the actual visits are getting shorter. Your take-home pay is smaller. Companies are now restricting who can join their insurance plans while continuing to pass on the high costs by reducing benefits, decreasing coverage, and increasing employees' out-of-pocket expenses.

Consequently, companies are increasingly shifting more of the responsibilities and costs for health care to employees, a trend similar to the restructuring that occurred with retirement and pension plans. A generation ago, employees had company-sponsored pension plans. They didn't need to worry about saving or investing for retirement because the company essentially promised its workers a monthly retirement pension. It was the company's job to ensure that it had enough money to pay its obligation. This arrangement became more costly as their retirees lived longer and increased in number. As a result, to stay competitive and cut costs, many organizations dispensed with their pension plans. Instead, they are providing 401(k) plans where the employees are ultimately responsible for determining whether they will have enough to retire.

Though most of us get health insurance through our employers, there is no legal obligation for them to provide that benefit. In the near future, most of us will have more responsibility regarding how we spend our money on staying healthy and getting the right treatment.

But the future is already here. To rein in costs, employers are now using "consumer-driven health plans" where you, not the insurance companies, get more control over how to spend your healthcare dollars. In January 2004, the government announced a new healthcare product known as the Health Savings Account, or HSA. Much less expensive than traditional comprehensive insurance plans, these plans have high deductibles. Like your auto insurance, these deductibles must be paid before the insurance company provides coverage. The premise is that as patients shoulder more financial responsibility through high-deductible insurance plans, they will seek health care more wisely.[5] In 2006, of the employers that offered health care benefits only 7 percent offered either plans with high deductibles or those that qualified to accompany a health savings account. Twelve percent of companies with more than 1,000 employees offered the plan.[6]

That figure is expected to continue to grow in the future, but employers have not adopted these products as quickly as first expected and neither have employees. Only 1 percent of the insured population currently has these accounts.[7] Perhaps this is not a big surprise after all — how confident are you of your ability to make the right choices when it comes to health care? Your health will rely not only on your ability to determine when to seek care but also on how much you can afford. If you don't spend wisely, you will pay more out of your own pocket than with the pricier comprehensive traditional plan. The next time your back aches and the sciatica flares up, you might wonder, with a high-deductible insurance plan, what to do. You could ignore the back pain and do nothing, see your primary care physician, or seek care with a back specialist, a spine surgeon.

Either physician might recommend additional testing like an x-ray, a CT scan, or an MRI. Since your insurance plan does not share the cost until your deductible is reached, did you save enough to pay for the doctors or any of these tests? Your back pain could be a common low back strain or a slow-growing cancer. What's your threshold to find out?

HSAs are an example of how our healthcare system is beginning to favor those with the knowledge of what tests, procedures, and medications are most appropriate and inexpensive. Although doctors are the most qualified to make these determinations, you are ultimately responsible for paying for the various medications, tests, and procedures. Soon only you will decide what you can and cannot afford. In the end, you, not an insurance company, will be rationing your own health care based on how much money you have.

Getting the best out of the American healthcare system relies on how well you choose the right insurance plan and the right physician. After you have picked the right team, the rest depends entirely on you. The more proactive and informed you are, the more likely you and your family will get the care you deserve.

You've already taken that first step by reading this insider's guide to ensure you have the best chance at achieving this goal. This book is divided into multiple sections. One section is devoted to the selection of the right insurance plan. We evaluate the pros and cons of HSAs as well as show you how you can find a high-quality insurance plan. There are dramatic differences between health insurance companies, and choosing the right one can prevent you from dying prematurely. For those who are uninsured, we talk about the importance of purchasing catastrophic medical insurance.

Unlike your home or your car, for which you must obtain insurance, there is no legal requirement to buy health insurance. But you are the most important financial asset that you own. With no insurance, you are gambling your future and your financial independence. Life happens. Medical care is extremely expensive. You can't will good health.

The second section of this book provides you with the tools to make the most out of your doctor visits. Remember, you need to be a wise patient. Wise patients are the ones who will most likely benefit from our current healthcare system. Wise patients are always prepared — they know what to ask, how to present themselves, and how to use their face time with the doctor wisely. Wise patients realize that their health is too precious, that having favorable health requires taking an active role, not just giving complete control to a doctor. The wise patient learns that the information he or she provides can make a doctor even better.

Learn which details are helpful to your doctor and remember what your doctor tells you (I give you an easy mnemonic device to help you do just that). Understand when you might want to have an establish visit with a new doctor and why a second opinion can be valuable. Familiarize yourself with the idea of informed consent; increasingly, you will need to decide between the benefits and risks of proposed medical procedures or tests offered by your doctor. Finally, learn when you don't need to see your physician.

In the third section, you will learn the prudent approach to staying healthy. Find out why the "annual physical" for healthy individuals under age fifty is obsolete and has no scientific or rational basis. Routine annual chest x-rays and urine tests are no longer, and have not been, the standard of care for over a decade. Once you know the preventive screening tests recommended by the American Cancer Society, the American Heart Association, and other organizations, only then will you know if you are getting the latest care. When problems are detected early, not only are they treated more easily, but they are also less costly both physically and financially.

The fourth section helps you find the right physician. A good physician not only possesses the knowledge to diagnose and treat you correctly and focuses on keeping you healthy, but also realizes that more and newer isn't necessarily better. Spending more doesn't promise better outcomes. To help you find a good doctor, you will learn how to verify board certification and state licensing, as well as understand the roles of other people you might interact with in the doctor's office like physician assistants and nurse practitioners.

In the fifth section I will focus on medications, which are a major financial burden for many. You will learn to understand the differences between generic and brand-name medications (and it isn't that generics are inferior because they are cheaper). You'll come to understand that you, as well as pharmaceutical representatives, can change your doctor's prescribing habits — and that might not be a good thing. Learn to ask your doctor the hard questions, like "Is this medication worth my money, or is all the advertising just that — hype?" Review websites that can help you choose inexpensive yet equally effective medications. To protect yourself from taking too much medication, learn how to decipher the over-the-counter medication package labeling. Finally, be comfortable in telling your doctor if a medication is too expensive. There are often alternatives.

In the sixth section I discuss the use of herbal and dietary supplements, body scans, and the trend of concierge physicians. Only until you understand these options thoroughly can you decide if they are worth your money.

The health care industry continues to come up with new ideas for how to deliver care more affordably with better outcomes. In the seventh section I discuss the fruits of some of these ideas: hospitalist physicians, patient group visits, and evidence-based medicine.

And in the last section I review how you can stay healthy by keeping active, maintaining a healthy weight, and finding a safe vehicle to travel in. I provide some suggestions for researching medical information from reputable sources using the Internet. I also share with you my thoughts about our healthcare system, which is in crisis.

Trying to get the most out of your money in health care is no more difficult than finding the best deal when purchasing a car. In many ways it is like a game. Once you know the rules, you will be more successful. By the end of this book, you will understand why you might consider enrolling in an HSA, particularly if you are healthy but still want health insurance; how to get the most out of your doctors appointments; know which tests you should demand to keep you healthy; understand how to find a high-quality physician; what the new trends in health care are and whether they are worth your money; and where to find trustworthy medical information on the Internet.

I should know. As a primary care physician employed by one of the top healthcare organizations in the United States, thousands of times a year I help my patients decide between different medications, tests, treatments, and therapies with the focus of keeping them healthy. As the only physician in my family, I never realized that my medical knowledge would be absolutely vital to ensure my family got the best care. Had I instead joined my classmates in the business world and not had medical training, I would be just like you, unsure if I was getting the best out of our healthcare system.

It shouldn't be that way. Ideally, our system would provide consistent high-quality care to all of us. Until there is a national urgency or strong leadership to re-invent our healthcare system, it is shaping up to favor not the patients who need it most, but those with the knowledge and the finances to get medical care. To stay healthy you need to plan and educate yourself. Your financial future depends on it. Your health depends on it. As a primary care physician, when I'm a patient, I'm ready for this new system. Are you? By the end of the book you will be.

But don't just take my word for it. Here's what others are saying:

> "Patients must take responsibility for their own care. They should seek information from trusted sources — such as their physicians, healthcare agencies specializing in their condition or disease (e.g., the American Diabetes Association), and organizations specializing in preventive care (e.g. the U.S. Preventive Services Task Force) — to learn what kind of preventive care or treatment they should be receiving, then work with their physicians to ensure that they get recommended care. Patients should not assume that their physicians will remember all that needs to be done. They can help their physicians provide good care by being active advocates for it."
>
> **— Conclusion of the RAND study (2004).**[8]

"There are widespread problems with the quality of much of America's health care. Although $1.2 trillion a year is spent on medical care, many people are receiving more care than they need, many are receiving less than they need, and many are receiving the wrong kind of care. In addition, preventable and harmful errors are occurring frequently. Millions of Americans are injured and tens of thousands die unnecessarily each year because of errors or the overuse, underuse, or misuse of services. Moreover, these problems are not being recognized or addressed adequately in this country today. We must find a better way to measure and improve quality."

— **National Coalition on Health Care (2003).**[9]

PART ONE:

The Most Important Policy You Will Ever Own

Thirty-seven percent of Americans are extremely or very confident that they possess enough knowledge to purchase health insurance on their own, which is comparable to feeling capable of investing their retirement savings without assistance.[10]

— 2006 Health Confidence Survey

"Your earning power is the single most valuable financial asset you control over your lifetime, more than your house or your investment portfolio."

— *Money* magazine, February 2006

Eighty-three thousand Americans die prematurely annually because they did not get care in accordance with guidelines from national expert committees and did not get the care backed by scientific evidence and research. Had they been enrolled in a high performing health insurance plan needless deaths would have been avoided.

— National Committee for Quality Assurance Report 2005

HEALTH INSURANCE, SAVINGS ACCOUNTS, AND COSTS

Why Now? Why Me? Do I Even Need Health Insurance?

What is the most valuable asset you own? Is it your car? Is it your house? Are your car and your house insured? Of course they are. Your car is insured because it is required by law. Your mortgage company or bank wouldn't give you money to purchase your home unless you could show proof of homeowner's insurance. In either case, should something happen to these important assets, you have some protection.

However, your most valuable asset is your health. Unlike in the previous examples, there is no law or requirement for you to protect it with health insurance.[11] Health insurance is completely optional. Though you might be able to wait to repair a car or have the dents and dings removed, the scenario is different with your health.

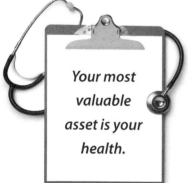

Your most valuable asset is your health.

You may not have the luxury of waiting if you are hurt, injured, or afflicted with an illness. Illness can be extremely expensive, especially if you don't have health insurance. Life happens. Disease happens. Protecting your most important asset, your health, is priceless. Healthy individuals can continue to work, make money, and support themselves and their families.

Amazingly, many people, including some of my family and friends, don't feel the need to purchase health insurance because they are healthy. Using the analogy of the house or car, I suppose if it wasn't required none of us would purchase auto or home owner's insurance either — since none of us expects to be in an auto accident or plans to be the victim of a burglary or house fire. Nevertheless, life happens. If you have good health, you can continue to make money and rebuild your life. On the other hand, if you become ill and are unable to regain your health, you can't provide for yourself or your family.

Consider the story of a twenty-four-year-old man, an uninsured, part-time waiter who was profiled on NBC's *Dateline*. Previously healthy, he never thought much of health insurance. Then he was seriously injured while traveling on the Staten Island Ferry. The October 2003 crash was the worst mass-transit accident in New York's history. The man required multiple surgeries, rehabilitation, physical therapy treatments, and medications. His total health care costs reached $213,000, which included x-rays ($2,700), medications ($13,000), various services ($15,000), ICU care ($15,000), and use of a semi-private room ($60,000).[12] In the end, he had some of his costs covered and enrolled in the state-funded Medicaid program for the poor.

Had he purchased health insurance, even a plan that only provided catastrophic coverage, his out-of-pocket expenses could have been capped at a few thousand dollars. Instead, he and his family face an enormous amount of debt.

Even if you believe that some people are simply unlucky, the odds are good that you will need health insurance to help treat a future illness. The American Cancer Society predicts that a man has a one in two chance and a woman a one in three chance of developing a cancer sometime during his or her lifetime. This calculation excludes patients with the more common forms of skin cancer like basal cell cancer and squamous cell cancer.

Understandably, Americans are reluctant to purchase health insurance as it is increasingly expensive and the benefit it provides is unclear. When surveyed, only 41 percent of Americans said that they were extremely or very confident that they knew enough to purchase health insurance on their own, which was much lower than the 78 percent who reported feeling confident in purchasing health insurance after talking to their doctor about health and health care. The survey found that choosing health insurance is as bewildering and scary as trying to figure out how to invest retirement savings on one's own. Only 40 percent felt confident doing so.[13]

Since 2000, premiums for family healthcare coverage have risen nearly 87 percent, much more rapidly than inflation (18 percent) and wage increases (20 percent).[14] In 2004, for the first time the national average for the total health care premiums paid to cover a family of four exceeded $10,000.

There are multiple reasons for this. Medical technology and therapies have improved so that patients who previously would have died from a heart attack or cancer are now surviving and living longer. Many consequently take prescription medications, often for life, and live long enough to develop another problem like an additional heart attack, stroke, or cancer. Newer treatments and medical devices while better than the past are also more expensive. As people live longer they also are more frail and require more resources and time with more medications, doctor visits, surgeries, and hospitalizations. Ironically, it is partially the success of medical science that has resulted in the current health care cost crisis.

> Of the over 45 million Americans who are uninsured, about 6.6 million earn household incomes of over $75,000.

Health insurance helps absorb some of the costs if you do need health care. In a 2004 Wall Street Journal Online/Harris Interactive Health-Care poll, nearly 2,400 Americans were asked to estimate the normal total cost, including what the patient and insurance company paid, for the following tests or services.[15] See what you think it is. The answers are in the take-home points at the end of this chapter.

> Blood work for cholesterol, blood sugar, or anemia.

> Hip replacement surgery (not including doctor fees, lab tests, and medication).

> A trip to the hospital to give birth by a C-section.

➤ A day and a night in a hospital (not including doctor fees, labs tests, and medication).

➤ A visit to a primary care doctor (not including lab tests or medication).

➤ A visit to a specialist (not including lab tests or medication).

Everyone should have some health insurance. Even if you cannot afford the traditional comprehensive health insurance, even a small amount of coverage may protect you from financial disaster. In 2004, a new insurance product, known as a Health Savings Account with a high-deductible plan, has made getting health insurance less expensive and provides protection from financial catastrophe. It is, however, not for everybody or for every situation.

Everyone should have some health insurance. Even if you cannot afford the traditional comprehensive health insurance, even a small amount of coverage may protect you from financial disaster.

CONSUMER-DRIVEN HEALTH PLANS (CDHPs), HEALTH SAVINGS ACCOUNTS (HSAs), AND PERSONAL RESPONSIBILITY

If you haven't already noticed, employers are offering more health insurance plans that are less comprehensive to lower their healthcare costs. As a result, you will now be faced with plans that require high deductibles before your insurance kicks in, much like your auto insurance. Some of these plans will be paired with Health Savings Accounts (HSAs), which allow workers to set aside money tax-free to pay for the deductible. These less traditional plans are collectively known as consumer-driven health plans (CDHPs). The theory is that employees will be more prudent about when to seek care and what prescription medications and tests to ask for when more of their own money is at stake.

Research already shows that participants in these plans are being more careful with their money. The majority take costs into account when seeking care as compared to a minority of enrollees in comprehensive health plans who do. But is looking at costs a good thing when deciding to get medical care? Given a chance, half of people enrolled in consumer directed health plans would be willing to switch insurance plans, as compared to only a third of participants in traditional plans. Participants in these plans were twice as likely to skip medical care over the past year due to cost and were likely to avoid, skip, or delay care when compared to those in traditional plans.[16,17] Perhaps it is not surprising that nearly twice as many participants in the comprehensive programs felt extremely or very satisfied with their plans (63 percent) as compared to those with high deductible plans (33 percent).[18]

What is the appeal, then, of CDHPs? Enrollees were attracted by the lower health care premiums as well as the chance to save money tax-free for future health care costs and retirement.[19]

It is unlikely that employers will be able to continue to offer robust comprehensive insurance plans as they are becoming too expensive. Reform from the government is equally unlikely, since the Health Savings Account is the cornerstone of the Bush Administration's answer to escalating health care costs. You will be seeing more of Health Savings Accounts in your future.

Here are some of the key features of the Health Savings Account:

➤ The HSA is portable and goes with you should you change employers. The account, like a 401(k) retirement plan, can be funded by the employee, the employer, or both, using tax-free dollars.[20]

➤ Like a 401(k) or IRA (individual retirement account), funds grow tax-free.

➤ Funds from the account can be spent on qualified medical expenses like doctor or dentist fees, prescription and nonprescription medications, eyeglasses or contact lenses, as well as hospital costs not covered by insurance.

➤ Unlike any other investment product available, funds go in tax-free, can grow tax-free, and are spent tax-free (on appropriate medical expenses) so that more of your hard-earned money goes to paying your medical expenses. Other investment accounts are always taxed at some point, are not allowed to be invested, or do not carry over the following year. For example, in a 401(k) or IRA, funds go in tax-free and grow tax-free, but when they are withdrawn, those funds are taxed. Dependent care (child care) expense accounts are funded using pre-tax dollars and are spent tax-free (on appropriate expenses), but cannot be invested and do not carry over to the next year. In other words, if you don't use it, you lose it. HSAs, however, do carry over to the following year. This allows you to build a larger account over time.

➤ Using pre-tax dollars, an employee's overall taxable gross income is also lowered, resulting in less tax owed to the government at the end of the year.

➤ HSAs must be linked to a high-deductible health insurance plan.

For healthy individuals, HSAs are a great way to save money. If you don't spend the money, it can be a great investment tool for retirement. That depends on how wisely you save and how well you stay healthy.

Before we continue about HSAs, let's go over some other important insurance terminology.

Types of Health Insurance Plans

➤ *Fee for Service.* With this type of health plan, patients can choose any provider who participates in the health plan (in the "network") and usually can see specialists without a referral. Physicians are paid based on the number of diagnoses and services performed. A preferred provider organization (PPO) is an example of a fee-for-service healthcare provider. Members of a PPO will have lower costs if they stay within the network of physicians designated by the insurance company. Obtaining services outside the network requires members to pay a larger portion of the costs. This freedom to select physicians comes at a cost, as PPO premiums are typically higher than HMO premiums. Enrollees of PPOs often have more problems with billing than HMO patients.[21]

➤ *Health Maintenance Organization (HMO).* Patients can only see providers in the HMO network. Members see specialists only after referral by the primary care doctor. The physicians are pre-paid to care for patients regardless of how little or how much they use the physicians. If you have not seen your doctor in the past two years, he gets paid a small monthly fee or "capitation" during that time. If you see him ten times this year, he gets the same fee. Members who choose to go outside of the HMO network have no insurance coverage and pay the entire medical cost. While HMOs generally cost less than PPOs, patients have less freedom and are restricted to selecting physicians within the HMO network

➤ *Point of Service (POS) plans.* Patients can choose to see physicians outside of the network. If referred by their doctor to an outside network provider, the insurance plan covers all or most of the bill. Usually, POS plans are attached as an option to HMO plans.

The difference between fee-for-service or PPO plans and HMO plans is very much like the experience of dining at an expensive restaurant and ordering off the menu. One option is you can order everything a la carte (PPO plan), create your own meal, and pay more. Another plan is to select from the prix fixe menu where you don't have as much choice, but can also have a good experience for less cost (HMO plan). In both cases, you had great service and excellent food. The quality of PPO and HMO plans are nearly identical, so the true difference lies in personal preference (complete freedom versus limited choices) and financial implications (differences in costs and dealing with billing).

Financial Terms

➤ *Deductible.* A deductible is just like the deductible you are familiar with from your auto insurance. The deductible is the amount you pay out of pocket before the insurance plan kicks in and starts paying your expenses. If the deductible is set low, the annual insurance premium is high, and vice versa. Deductibles can be as low as $500 and as high as $5,000 or more.

➤ *Co-insurance.* This refers to the percentage of the total cost that you are responsible for. For example, if an x-ray test costs $200 and you are responsible for 20 percent co-insurance, you need to pay $40, or 20 percent of $200.

➤ *Co-pay.* The fixed amount you need to pay for a service. A typical example is the office visit co-pay. You see your doctor and your co-pay is $10.

➤ *Pre-tax dollars.* The amount of money made or set aside before it is taxed by the state or federal government.

➤ *Post-tax dollars.* Money that has been taxed already by the state or federal government. Typically not subject to any additional income taxes.

> *The quality of PPO and HMO plans are nearly identical, so the true difference lies in personal preference (complete freedom versus limited choices) and financial implications (differences in costs and dealing with billing).*

Do I Qualify for an HSA?

You must be under sixty-five and enrolled in a high-deductible health insurance plan that meets the IRS requirements for an HSA. Your employer has probably already made sure your HSA options abide by those regulations. In 2005 for an individual, an HSA insurance plan must have an annual deductible ranging between $1,000 and $5,100. For a family, the limits are $2,000 to $10,200.[22] The actual number depends on the insurance plan you pick. The money used to fund the account is all in pre-tax dollars. This is exactly the same way you fund your 401(k) plan or dependent care account.

The amount you are allowed to put away in a year is determined by the deductible limit, IRS regulations, your age, and when you began your policy. If you started at the beginning of the year and it was 2006, you could put aside only the smaller amount of either the HSA deductible (between $1,050 to $5,250) or the IRS limit for an individual ($2,700 annually). For families, the choice again is between the smaller of the HSA deductible ($2,100 to $10,500) and the IRS annual limit for families ($5,450). For 2007, the limits were increased to $2,850 for an individual and $5,650 for a family. If you begin your HSA policy halfway through the year, the amount you are allowed to contribute is only half of that.

Enrollees fifty-five and older can contribute an additional $800 above the limit for 2007. For an individual, the maximum contribution in 2006 would be $3,400; for a family the total would be $6,150 if one spouse was fifty-five and older; and $6,850 if both spouses were fifty-five and older.

Due to legislation taking effect in 2007, individuals and families are now allowed to contribute to the full IRS limit even if their insurance deductible is smaller. The government will also allow a one-time transfer, tax-free, from an individual retirement account (IRA) to an HSA up to the HSA limit. With individuals and families allowed to put even more money in or take money from an

> *With individuals and families allowed to put even more money in or take money from an IRA to fund an HSA, it is clear that the government's strategy is to make sure that you have every opportunity to fund your own future health care costs.*

IRA to fund an HSA, it is clear that the government's strategy is to make sure that you have every opportunity to fund your own future health care costs.

Since limits and contributions will change periodically, much like the tax code, check with your tax advisor or accountant for the latest figures. You can also review Publication 969, *Health Savings Accounts and Other Tax-Favored Health Plans*, at www.irs.gov.

Any money you put aside can be spent on medical expenses tax-free. Withdrawals used on *non-qualified* medical expenses will not only require the account holder to pay taxes, but also an additional 10 percent penalty. If you wait until you are older than sixty-five, if you purchase items that are not qualified medical expenses, you only need to pay taxes. There is no additional 10 percent penalty.

Currently, health insurers provide HSAs, but banks, brokerage, and mutual fund companies will also offer HSA products and allow funds to be placed in interest-bearing and other accounts. Accountholders are often issued debit cards or checks to pay for their medical expenses. Debit cards are easier since these costs can be charged directly to the account. If the company that manages the HSA needs to reimburse you for writing personal checks to cover your expenses, you can expect to fill out paperwork

Because a high-deductible insurance plan is part of having an HSA, medical costs are not covered until you fulfill the deductible. So be prepared to pay more than you are used to if you need to get medical care.

But the upside is that plans with a high deductible cost less than traditional plans. Your monthly premiums are lower. As a result, your take-home pay should be higher. Using those extra dollars to fund your HSA, where monies can be contributed, withdrawn, and grown tax-free, lower your taxable income and can save you up to 30 percent on out-of-pocket medical costs.

What Are Qualified Expenses?

The IRS defines qualified medical expenses in Publication 502 and describes them as the "costs of diagnosis, cure, mitigation, treatment or prevention of disease, and the costs for treatments affecting any part or function of the body...Does not include expenses that are merely beneficial to general health, such as vitamins or a vacation."[23] Though medical expenses also include dental expenses, they do not include cosmetic procedures. You also cannot include expenses that were paid for by your insurance company.

Any of the following costs can be reimbursed with funds from the HSA.

> ➤ **Acupuncture**

> ➤ **Artificial Teeth**

> ➤ **Birth Control Pills**

> ➤ **Chiropractor**

> ➤ **Contact Lenses** — including the cleaning enzyme solution as well as the saline solution.

> ➤ **Dental Treatment** — including dental fees for x-rays and fillings, but not for teeth whitening.

> ➤ **Hospital Services** — including the costs of hospitalization, lodging, and meals (that are part of Inpatient medical care).

> ➤ **Medications** — both prescription and non-prescription.

You are, however, not obligated to use the money in the HSA for medical care. If you have reserved enough money elsewhere to cover your deductible, you can be more aggressive and treat the HSA like another retirement account.

A more comprehensive list is found in IRS Publication 502. Contact your HSA plan or your financial advisor if you need further clarification. Save your receipts!

Investment Options

With an HSA you will have the option to invest the funds in mutual funds or stocks to make even more money. Already, banks like JP Morgan Chase, Mellon Financial, Wells Fargo, and mutual fund companies like Fidelity have or will offer HSAs. As HSAs become more common, expect other companies to offer alternative investment choices to store your money.

Realize that the money you invest is for any future medical expenses and is expected to be used to cover that high deductible. Invest conservatively and carefully. Consider checking, savings, money market, or short-term bond funds that do not earn much interest, but will not cause you to lose your money.

You are, however, not obligated to use the money in the HSA for medical care. If you have reserved enough money elsewhere to cover your deductible, you can be more aggressive and treat the HSA like another retirement account. If you are young and don't plan on retirement for the next twenty years, investing in a stock or equity dominant fund might be a good option. If you aren't sure or are less interested in taking risks, put your money in short-term, intermediate bond funds that invest in government or respected companies. Consider investing in balanced mutual funds that allocate half the money in stocks and the other half in bonds. These funds are potentially less volatile than pure equity funds. Like most of us who witnessed the

If you plan on using the HSA as purely an investment/ retirement account, you must have funds elsewhere easily available for a rainy day.

stock market collapse of 2000 know, money invested in the market can quickly disappear.

This bears repeating. If you plan on using the HSA as purely an investment/retirement account, you must have funds elsewhere easily available for a rainy day. Investing in more aggressive plans may cause you to lose money, money you need for future health care costs. Our goal is to keep you healthy *and* financially savvy, not cause you to spend more money.

HSA Example

To understand everything you've learned so far, let's look at an example. Brian, thirty years old, compares a qualified high-deductible health plan and HSA with his previous, more comprehensive plan.

	New Health Plan with HSA	Old Comprehensive Health Plan
Deductible	$2400	$500
Monthly Premium	$89	$316
Annual Premiums	$1068	$3792
Total Savings	**$2724**	

With the HSA he saves over $2,700. Should he need medical care, he would need to pay $2,400 out of his pocket to cover his deductible before the plan provides coverage. He decides to fund a HSA with $1,000. This lowers his taxable annual income by $1,000 and saves him $280 if he is in the 28 percent tax bracket.

Starting in 2007, Brian can only fund his HSA up to either the HSA plan limit (in this case $2,400) or the IRS individual limit of $2,850.

	Account	No HSA Account
Total Income	$30,000	$30,000
Taxable Income	$29,000 ($30,000–1000)	$30,000
Income Tax Rate	28%	28%
Total Taxes	$8120	$8400
Tax Savings	**$280**	

So at the end of the year, Brian has saved $280 in taxes, owns a $1,000 HSA account that can grow tax-free, and has an additional $1,724 ($2,724 savings from premiums — $1,000 HSA) to spend on whatever he chooses. With the old plan all of his money went to pay for premiums.

But health care costs are more than just premiums. Let's look at other differences between the two health plans.

	New Health Plan with HSA	Old Comprehensive Health Plan
Prescription Medication Coverage	30% with network or non-network pharmacies after deductible reached. At network pharmacies, he receives the contracted rate.	$7 for generic drugs. $25 for formulary brand name drugs after $250 deductible. (30 day supply)
Doctor's Visits	30% with network providers. 50% with non-network providers.	$30 with network providers. 50% with non-network providers.

Continued on next page

	New Health Plan with HSA	Old Comprehensive Health Plan
Preventive Office Visit or Annual Physical Exam	$35 with network providers. Non-network providers not covered. 30% for Pap smear, mammogram, or immunizations.	$30 with network providers. Non-network providers not covered. Pap smear, mammogram, or immunizations included in the cost.
X-ray, Laboratory Tests	30% with network providers. 50% with non-network providers.	25% with network providers. 50% with non-network providers.
Pregnancy/ Maternity Care (outpatient)	30% with network providers. 50% with non-network providers.	25% with network providers. 50% with non-network providers.
Pregnancy/ Maternity Care (inpatient)	30% with network providers. 50% with non-network providers.	25% with network providers. 50% with non-network providers.
Physical Therapy	30% with network providers. 50% with non-network providers.	25% with network providers. 50% with non-network providers.

To keep your out-of-pocket costs low, you need to stay in your network. With health insurance, your network is the doctors, providers, and pharmacies that your insurance company has contracted with, identified, and preferred that you go to for care. Providers and pharmacies enter these contracts with the hope of getting more business. Insurance companies usually want a discount in return for sending more patients their way.

In both the HSA and comprehensive insurance plan there is a big price difference between selecting a network provider and a non-network provider. If you choose a network provider, you will pay a smaller amount for two reasons. First, there is a smaller co-insurance rate or percentage of the total fee that you are responsible for. Second, insurers usually negotiate with their network providers for a rate that's lower than what you'll pay for a non-network provider. Depending on the specifics of the plan, you might have no coverage at all for a non-network provider, which means you will be responsible for the entire bill. An office visit could easily be a couple of hundred dollars.

To keep your out-of-pocket costs low, you need to stay in your network.

This means that if the doctor is not in your network and you wish to continue care with him, it will cost you more despite having insurance. Doctors typically drop out of insurance plans because of problems or disagreements about reimbursement or reimbursement rates. Check the network list every year before you re-enroll for health insurance. Also consider whether the network of physicians and providers and the pharmacies' locations or hours are convenient for you. If not, you will spend more time and energy accessing your medical care.

Think of your network much like your bank's ATM network. While you can withdraw money out of any bank's ATM, you are typically charged more for accessing another bank's ATM instead of your own. You also can't deposit money into your account via another bank not in your network. If you select a bank with convenient ATM and bank locations, you will spend less time and energy getting to your account.

Consider Brian's choices. The difference between the HSA co-insurance payment with an in-network provider and the co-insurance payment with a comprehensive insurance plan differs by 5 percent. That might not be a lot. If you assume a physician's typical office visit is $100 with no insurance, the cost for the HSA plan would be $30 versus $25, a $5 savings. But as previously stated, Brian saved over $2,700 in premiums.

One of the big differences is how the two plans handle prescription drug coverage. With the old traditional comprehensive plan, Brian only pays $7 for generic medications. If he needs a brand-name medication, he first needs to fulfill a $250 medication deductible. Afterwards, he would only pay $25 for these drugs.

In the HSA plan, however, he has no prescription medication coverage and needs to pay full price until he has spent $2,400. After that amount has been reached, he begins to have some insurance coverage but will still need to pay 30 percent of his medication costs. If there is any good news, it's that his insurance company has negotiated for a lower price for medications. Although he still pays 100 percent of his medication costs until his deductible is fulfilled, he receives medications at the contracted rate.

Although the potential out-of-pocket costs vary between the two plans, the advantage with the HSA is that there is an opportunity to save money, particularly if you don't need health care. By setting money aside to fund the HSA, you lower your taxes. People with higher annual incomes and consequently higher taxes save even more. The trick is knowing how much to set aside for your account. While you do not lose the money, setting an amount too high "locks" it in for health care expenses. The money can be used for other expenses, but you must pay taxes and an additional 10 percent withdrawal penalty. But if you set the amount too low, you do not save as much in taxes and any other unpaid medical expenses will have to be paid out of pocket instead of from the HSA.

With the investment feature of the HSA, Brian might have ended the year with $1,000 and possibly more if he fully funded his HSA, did not use the healthcare system, and invested his money. Should he still have money in the HSA at age sixty-five, withdrawals for non-health care expenses would be taxed as income — but without the additional 10 percent penalty. Withdrawing money from an HSA at age sixty-five is no different than withdrawing money from a 401(k), an IRA, or other retirement account at that age. Therefore, if Brian chooses to use his

HSA merely as a retirement account, he can. He is under no obligation to pay for his healthcare expenses with the funds from his HSA.

Ultimately, with an HSA, Brian does not waste his hard-earned money on premiums, still has some healthcare protection from catastrophic events, and may even have an extra retirement account!

An HSA is a great option for patients who understand the extra tax benefit and how it increases the purchasing power of their money. The HSA also saves money on premiums. Consider an HSA if you feel comfortable with managing money, do not use the healthcare system frequently, and understand that you may pay more for medical services initially because of a higher deductible.

Spending Wisely

If you do qualify, are healthy, and are convinced that you can stay healthy and keep your money, you still need to know when to access the healthcare system and what to ask for. There is no point in becoming frugal and having large sums of money in your retirement accounts if you are not healthy enough or around long enough to enjoy it. Throughout the rest of this book, you will learn how to think like a doctor to get the most of your office visits, why "annual physicals" are not as important as targeted physical exams, which providers are best suited to handle your problems, and which healthcare trends are worth knowing about.

It's Not for Everyone

Even if you qualify for an HSA, there are situations where it makes sense to pay more in monthly premiums for a comprehensive health plan with little to no deductible. This is true especially if you anticipate a large medical expense. Skip an HSA if you are planning to have a baby, if you already have multiple chronic illnesses like heart disease, diabetes, or high blood pressure which requires daily medications, or if there is a fair chance you will be hospitalized or have surgery. These situations could easily cost thousands of dollars, wiping out any potential savings in increased take-home pay and perhaps even your own personal accounts.

If Brian is married and he and his wife are trying to have a baby, they will need to know that a normal vaginal delivery can cost anywhere from $6,000 to $10,000. A C-section can cost between $10,000 and $15,000. Some HSA plans have no coverage for any prenatal office visits or hospitalization costs to have a baby. Others will require that the high deductible be fulfilled first; afterwards, only a percentage of the costs (co-insurance) need to be paid by the patient. So remember, an HSA is not the perfect plan for all situations.

It is still, however, better than going without any insurance. One young couple who lost their health insurance decided to go without, even though they were expecting a baby. Though they could have purchased an individual policy for $525 a month with a $2,500 deductible, they gambled, thinking it would be cheaper to simply pay for the delivery out of pocket. Unfortunately, the mother required an emergency cesarean delivery and even after emptying their individual retirement saving accounts and getting the hospital to lower its charges, they owed the hospital over $10,000. Now they may be forced to sell farm land that has been in the family for over thirty years.[24] Realize that if you choose an HSA and then develop a serious medical problem like cancer, heart disease, or diabetes, you may not be able to switch back to a comprehensive health insurance plan in the future. You may be stuck with the HSA for good — so choose wisely.

> *Realize that if you choose an HSA and then develop a serious medical problem like cancer, heart disease, or diabetes, you may not be able to switch back to a comprehensive health insurance plan in the future. You may be stuck with the HSA for good — so choose wisely.*

Whatever you choose, remember that life happens and your health is not certain or predictable. *Protect your health and your wealth — get health insurance coverage.*

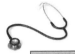 **Real-Life Example**

> When one of my patients became a father for the second time, the last thing on his mind was the financial protection provided by his medical insurance. His wife's pregnancy was uneventful. The delivery went smoothly. His new son appeared healthy and the parents were eager to take him home. But hours before discharge, an astute pediatrician detected a heart murmur, and to be on the safe side ordered an echocardiogram (heart ultrasound).
>
> Within a couple of weeks, my patient's son underwent open-heart surgery to correct a congenital heart defect. The total cost of care was $250,000. While my patient was ready to sell his home to save his baby, his health insurance covered all of it. He had the traditional comprehensive coverage where there was no deductible.

Since HSAs need to be linked to a high-deductible medical plan, you first need to fulfill the deductible before the insurance company will begin to pick up the tab. Even then, you will face larger co-insurance payments and co-pays as compared to a traditional comprehensive plan. You might still save money if you don't need health care often, as these high-deductible plans usually have lower premiums. These high-deductible plans are designed to protect you from catastrophic financial losses so that you won't become bankrupt in order to get the care you or your loved ones need.

THE QUALITY OF YOUR HEALTH
INSURANCE PLAN MATTERS!

> "Patients must take responsibility for their own care…
> seek information from trusted sources…learn what
> kind of preventive care or treatment they should be
> receiving, then work with their physicians to ensure
> that they get recommended care. Patients should not
> assume that their physicians will remember all that
> needs to be done. They can help their physicians pro-
> vide good care by being active advocates for it."
>
> — **Conclusion of the RAND study (2004).**[25]

Saving money is particularly rewarding when you manage to purchase a superior product at a good price. Take the experience of buying
a car. While on the surface all cars provide you with transportation,
some cars are more popular than others and some cars are also safer
than others. You'll pay more for a higher-quality car. You should take
the same approach with buying health insurance, as all health insurance
plans are not created equal.

Unlike other products and services we purchase, it is difficult for
consumers to adequately determine whether a health insurance plan is
worth their hard-earned dollars. As a result, many of us choose plans
based on their cost, or on whether or not our doctors participate in the
plan. However, this choice could cost you your life.

Within the United States, medical treatment for the same disease
varies dramatically, with major consequences to the patient. Take the
case of heart attack patients. There is clear scientific evidence that the
addition of a beta blocker heart medication decreases the risk of future

heart problems. Although taking this medication is currently considered the standard of medical care, less than 50 percent of heart attack patients in Mississippi receive this life-saving drug. In Massachusetts on the other hand, nearly every heart attack patient is taking it. The issue is not related to physician compensation or the ability to pay for medication, since all the patients received the same insurance, Medicare.[26] Ultimately, the issue stemmed from whether the doctors were consistently following the guidelines established by the American Heart Association.

Within the United States, medical treatment for the same disease varies dramatically, with major consequences to the patient.

Once established, these guidelines or "best practices" can take up to a decade to be implemented by a majority of healthcare practitioners. *A review of 20,000 patients from 12 metropolitan areas showed that only 76 percent of breast cancer patients, 73 percent of pre-natal patients, 69 percent of low back pain patients, 68 percent of coronary heart disease patients, and 65 percent of high blood pressure patients received the recommended care developed by expert medical committees.*

Over a third (36 percent) of elderly patients did not receive the pneumonia vaccine, which would have prevented 10,000 deaths annually. And another 68,000 lives could have been saved if the remaining 35 percent of high blood pressure patients had received appropriate treatment. Experts reflected that this study should not be "read as an indictment of physicians or nurses. They are simply working in a care system that is incapable of supporting excellence, a system we have designed for failure."[27]

The National Committee for Quality Assurance (NCQA), which evaluates health insurance plans, estimated that in 2005, as many as 83,000 Americans died prematurely not because of hospital errors, misdiagnoses, or negligence, but because they did not get care in accordance with guidelines from national expert committees, and they did not get the care backed by scientific evidence and research.[28] In high quality health plans, simple factors like controlling high blood pressure, lowering cholesterol, and managing diabetes to the recommended levels get done and needless hospitalizations and deaths are averted.

When NCQA compared the performance of the top 10 percent of health plans with the national average on measures like screening for breast cancer, advising patients to quit smoking, and offering immunizations for flu shots, they discovered variability among plans exceeding 20 percent. Using similar criteria to compare the safety performance of the top 10 percent of airline carriers with the national average, the quality gap was far less than *1 percent.* The same applied for banking and manufacturing. How safe would you feel about flying if among the various airlines there was a quality variance of over 20 percent? Yet when it comes to health care, consumers don't appear to be aware or concerned.

An additional frightening fact is that only a small number of health plans, which enroll about 25 percent of insured Americans, submitted their performance data for NCQA review. This means there is a very good chance that your health plan could do better, particularly if it is not listed on the NCQA website.

Although there is great variability on the type of care you receive, based on where you live or on which insurance plan you choose, there are health insurance plans and programs that consistently deliver high quality care.

Now that you know this, begin your search for a high-quality health plan by doing the following:

> ➤ Refer to the NCQA website at www.ncqa.org to research insurance plans. PPOs, HMOs, Medicare, and Medicaid programs are rated on access and customer service; the providers; programs provided by the plan to improve and/or maintain health; and services in place

to help those members with chronic illnesses like diabetes and asthma. Fortune 500 companies, state, and federal governments use NCQA report cards to determine which health insurance plans to offer their employees.

➤ Review *U.S. News & World Report's* ranking on health plans, which was developed with NCQA, at www.usnews.com/healthplans.

➤ Check out *Consumer Reports,* which periodically ranks health plans. Visit their website at www.consumerreports.org.

➤ Do your research. If you have a chronic illnesses like diabetes, asthma, congestive heart failure, or emphysema, does the insurance plan have programs specifically designed for you to improve your overall health and quality of life?

➤ Also, find out whether the plan promotes wellness and preventive health. Health plans that have low to no co-payments for screening tests like mammograms or Pap smears, preventive interventions like immunizations and annual physicals, are probably promoting good health.

➤ Look at the plan's provider network — the number of participating physicians and affiliated hospitals available to choose from. The physician's office and hospital closest to you may not necessarily take your insurance plan, so check first.

Your chance of getting the best and latest care may rely more on the insurance plan than on the individual physician, particularly when it comes to common diseases like diabetes, heart disease, high blood pressure, and cancer.

There are many existing high-quality healthcare systems designed for excellence. Researching and selecting such plans can improve the likelihood that you receive the latest recommended care.

The importance of the quality of the insurance plan cannot be understated. Your chance of getting the best and latest care may rely more on the insurance plan than on the individual physician, particularly when it comes to common diseases like diabetes, heart disease, high blood pressure, and cancer. The *Wall Street Journal* reported that many health insurance plans, and plan purchasers like General Motors and Ford Motor Company, are promoting a pay for performance system in which physicians are paid bonuses for offering simple but proven interventions like preventive screening, immunizations for appropriate patients, and treating diabetics and others with chronic illness to the level recommended by expert medical committees. These treatments may be costly initially, but pay dividends later.

Here are two examples of how a small change in an incentive for doctors resulted in better physician care. For years, the standard of care for heart failure patients has been the use of an ACE inhibitor medication. The addition of the medication has been shown to prolong patient survival. Yet in one study, only 40.8 percent of patients were prescribed this medication. Once financial incentives were introduced, however, the percentage of patients on the medication increased to 64.2. In another instance, the percentage of diabetic patients who were offered the HgbA1c blood test, used to determine how well controlled a patient's blood sugar is, increased from 51.5 percent to 79.6 percent once a financial incentive was offered to physicians.

The quality of your insurance plan can also affect the likelihood that you will get needed care. For example, another report found that patients enrolled in low-ranked HMOs or PPOs had twice as much difficulty obtaining the care they needed as compared to patients enrolled in high-ranked plans. With a low-ranked plan, not only could it be harder to get the care you need, but when you receive it, it might not be the most cutting edge.

Besides considering NCQA accreditation when you look at insurance plans, also consider the plan's non-profit or for-profit status. If given a choice between two equally qualified health plans, you will probably do best to choose the plan run by a non-profit company. Publicly traded, for-profit companies may have a different agenda and be more concerned about their stockholders than their patients. Some of these companies, for example, are reinstating unpopular restrictions and cutting benefits as a way of curtailing costs.[29]

But consistency and providing the latest care doesn't just fall to physicians and health plans. Hospitals are also being scrutinized. Recently, Medicare made available to patients information about the quality of service provided at many institutions. In 2005, the agency published quality of care data on hospitals that treat heart attacks, congestive heart failure, and pneumonia.[30] They found that only 39 percent of hospitalized patients with pneumonia receive the recommended care.

To help ensure the correctness of this data and an accurate reporting sample, Medicare has instituted a financial incentive to hospitals, for whom reporting is voluntary. Medicare plans to decrease reimbursements to hospitals that choose not to report. It is hoped that this will encourage more hospitals to participate in quality-of-care surveys, and that patients and health plans will use this information to determine which hospitals provide the best care.

A great tool to evaluate hospital performance can be found at www.leapfroggroup.org. The Leapfrog Group is an organization of healthcare purchasers whose goal is to improve patient safety, healthcare quality, and affordability by rewarding and recognizing healthcare providers that perform well. Their website rates hospitals in terms of their success at implementing safeguards, processes, and systems, as well as on their ability to maximize patient outcomes. Objectively assess hospital performance the same way you would research other big ticket purchases. There is, after all, nothing bigger or more important than your health.

Quality matters. But you can only benefit from the care offered by high-quality programs and hospitals by taking time to do research. Once you've done your homework, pick a quality plan during open enrollment. If your employer does not offer a highly ranked program, you can still ensure you receive the latest in health care. Subsequent sections of this book will help you understand what you need to do to maximize your chances for good health.

DO YOUR HOMEWORK. QUESTION EVERYTHING AND PAY NOTHING (RIGHT AWAY)

In college, my brother had a terribly painful sore throat. Far from home, he called my parents, who called their insurance company for advice on what to do and who to see. He ended up seeing a doctor employed by the student health department, who then referred him to an otolaryngologist (a head and neck surgeon, in the past known as an ear, nose, and throat specialist) to provide further care.

A couple of months later, the insurance company billed my parents $140: $20 for the first physician and $120 for the specialist. My mother immediately called to dispute the charges and wrote a follow-up letter. Prior to my brother's appointments, she had called the insurance company to ask about coverage, approval, and payment. She was told that his doctor visits would all be covered. During these calls she wrote down the names of the representatives she talked to, the dates and times, and included these facts in her subsequent phone calls and letter. In the end, the insurance company paid the bills and covered the disputed charges.

The lesson is that you should always check your medical bills thoroughly. Billing errors do occur. According to the AMBR, a medical-bill auditor, 85 percent of hospital bills contain errors.[31] When my mother needed breast cancer treatment, some of her physicians billed her afterwards even though she paid her co-pay. One doctor's office claimed that her insurer denied the billing charges and that she was responsible for the difference. She called the insurance company, reviewed the itemized list, and discovered that the insurer had paid for the service, but it was grouped together under one charge. Although the doctors didn't like the contracted reimbursement, the services they provided were included in the lump sum and so no additional money needed to be paid.

When my father needed the services of a new specialist, my mother called the insurance company to make sure his doctor was in their network. Although he did participate in my parents' health plan, the payment for the office visit was denied by the insurance company. The billing department had requested payment using the medical group's corporation name, which was not on file, instead of the individual physician's name. This happened twice. Fortunately, each time my mother was able to rectify the problem. The charges were completely covered, and my parents didn't need to pay any more fees.

Scrutinize your medical bills as carefully as your monthly credit card statements, grocery bills, or anything else you buy regularly. Two things can happen with insurance denials. The physician's office resubmits the paperwork correctly or will ask the patient for the difference. If a charge is denied, do not pay it immediately. Call the insurance company and see what happened. Call your doctor's office and speak to the office or business manager to clarify the situation. Only pay what you are supposed to pay. Do not worry how this might affect the care from your physician. They may not know all the details and intricacies of medical billing or the specifics of individual patients' accounts. (There is a reason they hire business managers — so they can focus on taking care of you.) Ultimately, it is your responsibility to make sure that simple mistakes do not prevent you from getting the coverage you paid for. It is, after all, your money.

Unless it is a true medical emergency, check briefly with your insurance plan before you seek care. Inquire about how to deal with urgent and non-urgent problems when traveling away from home. Health insurance plans contract with certain pharmacies, laboratories, and radiology offices to receive your medications, draw your blood, or take your x-rays, and may change their contracts periodically. In a perfect world, all laboratories, pharmacies, and other medical services would accept everyone's insurance plan. Fortunately, many accept most insurance plans; just be sure you are not the exception.

In a real emergency, call 911 or go to the nearest emergency room. In situations like these, it is always better to deal with the medical problem first and insurance coverage later.

Finally, to save even more money, keep your bills and receipts. The IRS allows you to deduct your medical bills if they exceed 7.5 percent of your adjusted gross income. While it won't lower your medical costs, it might lower your taxes.

YOU'RE ON YOUR OWN

Recently Lost Job and Consolidated Omnibus Budget Reconciliation Act (COBRA)

Enacted in 1986, the Consolidated Omnibus Budget Reconciliation Act (COBRA) is a federal law that allows you to continue your employer's group health insurance coverage at the group rate if you have left the company for another job that does not provide health insurance, become part-time without health insurance, or are unemployed.

The good news is that with COBRA you get the cheaper group rate. This is particularly valuable if your medical history contains serious problems like cancer and heart disease, for which individual coverage is extremely expensive. Unfortunately, the bad news is that you pay both your original contribution as an employee as well as the much larger employer's contribution. The average yearly group rate premium would be $3,383 for an individual and $9,068 for a family. Under COBRA, these costs are completely borne by the employee — compared with $508 for an individual and $2,412 for a family if the employer were subsidizing the premium.

If you can afford the higher premium, you can continue coverage with COBRA for up to eighteen months. In special situations coverage can be extended to thirty-six months. However, COBRA does not apply to companies with less than twenty employees covered in a group health plan, workers who are covered by federal government plans or church plans, and those enrolled in individual insurance plans. To learn more about COBRA, go to the U.S. Department of Labor website at www.dol. gov/ebsa/faqs.

Between Jobs/Recent College Graduate

Although COBRA allows individuals and families to purchase coverage at group rates, for healthy people an individual plan, while less comprehensive, is typically less expensive. Recent college graduates or those in between jobs should consider short-term health insurance. You can research individual or short-term insurance plans at www.ehealthinsurance.com.

Patients with pre-existing conditions (histories of cancer, diabetes, or coronary artery disease, for example) or those who require multiple prescription medications may find individual plans too expensive even with minimal coverage and should opt for the group coverage through COBRA. Another option is to consider working part-time for an employer that provides benefits. Companies like Starbucks, UPS, Costco, and Whole Foods Market provide health insurance to part-time employees.[32] With increasing health care costs, these firms are becoming the exception rather than the norm.

HEALTH CARE COSTS — HOW MUCH DOES IT COST FOR PROCEDURES AND TESTS?

An aspiring film director and soon-to-be college graduate, my brother has been lamenting how low his future earnings will be. Not surprisingly, like many people I meet, my brother is considering not purchasing any health insurance in order to save money. He figures that since he's healthy his money could be better spent elsewhere rather than on a costly insurance plan.

Hopefully when he graduates he will, at a minimum, enroll in a high-deductible plan or even seek temporary coverage, until he finds a job with benefits. If a high-deductible plan is still too expensive, he should find an insurance broker and purchase catastrophic health insurance. Although it won't cover any office visits or emergency room visits, it would protect him from going bankrupt if he were to require prolonged hospital stays or surgery. Health insurance is the only way to preserve his dream.

Many examples point to the importance of insurance coverage. Life happens. Take the case of the fifty-seven-year-old uninsured rental property owner who fell off a ladder while repairing his rental property roof. While he was able to go back to work, his wife, just to be sure, called an ambulance. After a trip to the emergency room which resulted in x-rays of his chest, pelvis, and knee, as well as a CT scan, he was sent home. No problems were found. Later, he received a bill of $15,000, more than half of his annual income.[33] Hospitals, trying to cover costs, are charging uninsured patients up to four times more than insured patients.[34]

> *The odds are good that in the future you will need medical care, even if you are healthy.*

The odds are good that in the future you will need medical care, even if you are healthy. Every year about one in six men develops prostate cancer and one in seven women is diagnosed with breast cancer. In the fall of 2003, my mother became one of those women diagnosed with breast cancer. She required breast surgery, chemotherapy, and radiation treatments. The cost for the chemotherapy medications alone (four treatments of Taxol at $2,000 each and $1,300 worth of treatments of adriamycin, cytoxan, and aloxi) would have cost $13,200. Add to that figure the costs of the office visits (not the co-pay), the additional lab tests, equipment (like IVs), medications, x-rays, and nursing costs, and the price for her illness would have been exorbitant to pay out of pocket.

Not convinced? Consider that in 2001, 80 percent of Americans made at least one trip to a healthcare provider, emergency room, or to a pharmacist to fill a prescription medication.[35] If you still don't think you need health insurance, at least look at some of the figures below. These figures are probably now even higher as medical costs continue to rise.

80 percent of Americans made at least one trip to a health-care provider, emergency room, or to a pharmacist to fill a prescription medication.

The cost of...

A typical hospital room:	$3,000 or more per day
Monitored heart unit room:	$3,800 or more per day
Intensive Care Unit (ICU):	$6,200 or more per day
CT scan of the head:	$1,400
MRI of the abdomen:	$2,100
X-ray of knee (two views):	$75 to $150
MRI of the knee:	$775 to $1,500
Physical therapy visit:	$70 to $150
Open-heart bypass surgery:	$73,000 to $110,000
Lithotripsy (shockwave treatment for kidney stones):	$18,000
Hip replacement:	$11,390 to $22,860[36]

These charges do not include the costs of additional medications, IVs, laboratory tests, or x-rays ordered by the physicians caring for you. Doctor fees are also not included in the above rates. Just one bad car accident requiring hospitalization, even for observation, could easily cost you thousands of dollars.

Having health insurance protects you from being overcharged.

Realize that health care when you don't have insurance actually costs more. According to the Centers for Medicare and Medicaid Services, the national average charge for a hernia surgery is $16,310, while the average payment by the insurer was only $4,991.[37] The charge for a heart valve replacement was $115,221, while the reimbursement was $38,528. Having health insurance protects you from being overcharged.

Do not expect the federal program Medicaid to automatically come and assist you, either. Having low income is only one criterion. Eligible Medicaid recipients are defined by federal and state statute. Typical enrollees include children under age six who live in a family with an annual income below 133 percent of the federal poverty level (which in 2007 for a family of four was $20,650 for the 48 contiguous states); a pregnant woman with the same annual income limits; and individuals who qualify for a state's Aid to Families with Dependent Children (AFDC) program.[38]

Because in order to be a candidate for federal assistance you must prove that you are destitute, individuals will sometimes divorce their spouses or transfer or liquidate all their assets. I've seen families agonize over the decision to spend their life savings to pay for medical care, knowing they will have nothing left — but will qualify for Medicaid. I've witnessed devoted spouses adamantly refuse to divorce just for the sake of getting assistance. These are heart wrenching experiences. Do not let them happen to you.

If you have limited resources, protect yourself from catastrophic losses by buying health insurance with high deductibles and low premiums. Protect your financial health until you can enroll in more comprehensive coverage. It might seem like a waste of money: you don't smoke, don't drink, exercise regularly, and don't ever expect to need health insurance. You simply don't get sick. Unfortunately, however, life and good health are somewhat unpredictable. How do you know if and when one of your skin cells will become a melanoma? How sure are you that another driver on the freeway won't cut you off or even be inebriated and cause a serious, but not fatal, accident? One study suggested that the number of deaths incurred because people who didn't have health insurance was as high as 18,000 people annually — roughly the name number of people dying from diabetes.[39]

One study suggested that the number of deaths incurred because people who didn't have health Insurance was as high as 18,000 people annually — roughly the name number of people dying from diabetes.

Unless you live life in a bubble, stuff happens. I see it every day in my practice. When I had a two-month gap between my residency program and my new job, the first thing I did was call an insurance agent and purchase catastrophic healthcare coverage to protect myself. Because you never know.

Protect your health and protect your finances. Insure yourself and your family. Get the best possible health insurance coverage you can afford.

TAKE-HOME POINTS

✓ **The most valuable asset you own is your health.** Life happens. Disease happens. You need to protect your health the same way you protect your car and your home — purchase insurance.

✓ **Purchasing health insurance, even plans that provide only minimal coverage, can prevent catastrophic financial losses.** Comprehensive coverage is becoming more expensive and employers will continue to shift more costs to employees through consumer-driven health plans. These changes also affect current and future retirees.

✓ **When comparing health plans, first see what options are offered by your employer.** Determine whether you prefer the flexibility of choosing your own doctors as well as the burden of paperwork and billing found in PPO plans or the closed networks of HMO plans. Regardless of the plan, research consumer advocacy magazines and the NCQA to ensure that you have a high-quality health plan. Remember, it is your health and your money.

✓ **If you're healthy, a Health Savings Account (HSA) is a great way to save money on healthcare expenses.** You must be under sixty-five and enrolled in a qualified high-deductible health insurance plan. The advantages of the HSA include lower taxes, the ability to use 100 percent of your earned dollars toward medical expenses, the freedom to let your money grow tax-free, and maintaining possession of the account regardless of your job situation. Savings of up to 30 percent are possible.

✓ **Ask questions about your medical bills.** Call your insurance company if you think some itemized charges should be covered. Discuss the charges with your physician's office manager if you feel the office made an error. This should not compromise the care you receive.

✓ **Remember that you get what you pay for.** There is no free lunch. A plan with a low premium and a high deductible means that when you need health care, you must have enough money to cover any future healthcare expenses up to the deductible. This can range anywhere from hundreds to thousands of dollars. Only then do the co-insurance benefits begin. A high premium and a low- or no-deductible plan means you need to set aside less money, but you are often paying significantly more per month in premiums.

✓ **How did you do on the poll?** Here are the answers: $300 for blood work, $25,000 for hip surgery, $13,500 for a C-section, $3,600 for a day and night hospital stay, $80 for a primary care office visit, and $550 for an ambulance trip. Are these costs greater than you expected?

PART TWO:

Mastering the Ten-Minute Doctor Office Visit

Twenty-three seconds: that's the average amount of time a doctor waits before interrupting a patient.

Wise patients know that staying healthy and getting better sometimes means a trip to the doctor's office is necessary. But they realize that they don't live in an ideal world, and there are many obstacles that may prevent them from getting the most out of their visit — including inadequate face time with the doctor. To overcome this challenge, the wise patient prepares for the encounter.

Twenty-three seconds. That's the average amount of time a doctor waits before interrupting a patient. In fact, one study showed that nearly 70 percent of the time physicians interrupted patients in the first fifteen seconds of the visit.[40] If that isn't bad enough, other research indicates that the actual visit and face to face time with a doctor is less than twenty minutes.[41] If you feel like you're getting rushed through the office visit, you're right.

One reason for these short visits stems from the way physicians are currently compensated. Insurance companies pay doctors for the number of diagnoses and services provided to enrollees. This is where the phrase "fee for service" originated. As a result, doctors get paid more to *do* more. Physicians can increase their compensation by seeing more

The most important tool available to doctors is the ability to take an accurate and comprehensive patient history.

patients and/or doing more medical procedures. With insurance reimbursement rates decreasing and with physician offices' overhead, supplies, and staff expenses increasing despite you paying higher health insurance premiums, the ability to get more by doing more is important. In a typical work day, a primary care doctor may see twenty to thirty patients. If you sign up for a PPO health insurance plan, your doctor definitely participates in a fee-for-service system.

With the reality of shorter office visits and high patient volume, wise patients and doctors know that the most important tool available to doctors is the ability to take an accurate and comprehensive patient history. Even today, understanding a patient's symptoms and medical history provides physicians with the critical information they need to begin their initial assessment and formulation of a treatment plan. The next step could include beginning treatment, requesting additional tests, or referring to another physician.

THE IMPORTANCE OF A MEDICAL HISTORY

Before medical students examine their first real patients, they spend months refining their listening and interviewing skills. Listening carefully and asking important questions often points toward a diagnosis.

At times, however, a diagnosis is elusive. Either the disease is uncommon and requires more investigation or the patient is unable to provide the pertinent facts or information to help clarify the problem. In both situations additional tests and procedures are usually ordered. Uncommon illnesses can take time to diagnose, but if you provide your doctor the relevant information he needs, you may minimize unnecessary tests and costs. Even with the available advanced medical technology, a good history that supplies the necessary information is a superior tool and helps doctors reach a diagnosis more quickly.

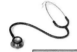 ## Real-Life Example

I had known Mr. Sanchez for years. When he talked, he was forced to pause every couple of sentences to catch his breath. His pudgy and wrinkly elderly face was a consequence of both his periodic use of prednisone to help calm his emphysema and years of prolonged sun exposure and smoking.

But on this day, Mr. Sanchez's visit had nothing to do with his breathing. He was suffering from severe abdominal pain and had been to the emergency room twice. Both times, the diagnosis was unclear. He was told he *might* have passed a kidney stone, but when I greeted Mr. Sanchez he was still in excruciating pain.

During his first emergency room evaluation he had a CT scan of the abdomen. It did not show a kidney stone or any other abnormalities with his internal organs that could explain his symptoms. He returned a couple of days later, still in severe pain. Another evaluation was done and an abdominal x-ray still did not reveal anything.

I asked Mr. Sanchez to tell me his story and relay the symptoms he had noticed before going to the emergency room. He complained of sudden, severe pain radiating from the low back to the front of the lower abdomen. He had no fever. The pain caused him to be extremely nauseated and was a lot worse when he lay down. Only when he sat upright or stood up did the pain improve slightly.

While the location and severity of the pain could have been caused by a kidney stone, changing positions would generally not affect the intensity of the pain. He also denied seeing any blood in the urine. These symptoms weren't entirely consistent with a kidney stone.

I asked him some other questions. When did his symptoms start? What had he been doing that day? He related a typical quiet retiree's day: he got up, ate breakfast, and read the paper. Nothing out of the ordinary occurred — except that he did, however, flip his mattress that morning. The pain seemed to come on shortly after that.

This additional information led me to believe that his pain could have been caused by a nerve being pinched by a cracked vertebral bone in the spinal column of his back. While normally the bones in the back are quite strong, his use of prednisone over the years could have weakened them. A broken vertebral bone would explain why the pain was worse when lying down. And the pinched nerve would refer pain from the back to the front of the abdomen, where he felt it most.

Mr. Sanchez was exquisitely sensitive when I pushed on his spine. An x-ray of the spine showed a collapsed vertebral bone due to osteoporosis. With the correct diagnosis, Mr. Sanchez was given strong narcotic medications, started on treatment for osteoporosis, and told to expect his symptoms to slowly get better over the next six to eight weeks. At a follow-up appointment, Mr. Sanchez felt better and had no more back pain or abdominal pain.

To get the most out of an office visit, you need to be a good and effective storyteller. While the previous example showed how a physician can get the information that he wants, it also shows that when the physician does not dig deeper into the patient's medical history (note that Mr. Sanchez had been to the emergency room twice), *the lack of information can result in additional testing and work-ups that may not lead to the correct diagnosis.*

Providing enough information for your doctor — even if he doesn't seem to have enough time — is simply a matter of telling your story in a way that your doctor can understand. Once your physician has a clear idea of your symptoms, concerns, and expectations, he can begin a treatment plan to get you feeling better and to keep you healthy. By delivering your story using language the doctor understands, you might figure out the reasons for your own problem or symptoms.

PROVIDING THE PERFECT HISTORY

Before we discuss how to give the perfect history, let's look at two patients who see their doctor for the same problem.

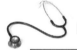 **Example One: Typical Patient A**

> **Doctor:** What brings you in today?
>
> **Patient:** Well, Doctor, I've been feeling really tired over the past month. I don't feel like my usual self. I just feel really tired and I don't feel good.
>
> **Doctor:** Hmmm. Anything else?
>
> **Patient:** No, that's it.
>
> **Doctor:** I see…what else have you noticed?
>
> **Patient:** Nothing else. I'm exercising regularly and sleeping well. But I feel like I can doze off at any time. I try to take good care of myself. I take vitamins. I haven't changed anything. I don't get it.

Doctor: So what makes your fatigue better or worse?

Patient: I'm not sure, I'm just really tired.

Doctor: Do you feel tired in the morning when you get up or more at the end of the day?

Patient: I've never paid much attention. I just know I don't have any energy.

Doctor: Have you had any weight loss or gain?

Patient: No.

Doctor: Any problem with your appetite? Are you eating regularly? Skipping meals?

Patient: I haven't had any problems.

Doctor: Do you feel depressed or stressed?

Patient: No. What do you think it is?

This conversation might continue for many minutes or the doctor, feeling rushed for time, might proceed to an exam, order tests, or write a prescription.

Look at the same example with the wise patient below.

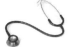

Example Two: Wise Patient

Doctor: What brings you in today?

Patient: Well, Doctor, I've been feeling really tired over the past month. I don't feel like my usual self.

Doctor: Hmmm. Anything else?

Patient: I've been really tired, mostly at the end of the day. I feel like I might doze off and I have really low energy. I'm sleeping well and have no problems with eating. I haven't noticed any weight loss or gain. No fever, cough, or cold symptoms. I just feel really

> sluggish. Nothing much has changed in my life. I
> still exercise regularly and take vitamins. I don't feel
> depressed or stressed. But I feel completely wiped
> out when I come home from work. I eat regularly.
> Haven't changed my diet. I did notice that when I
> started feeling tired that it was the same time my job
> got a lot busier. What do you think it is?

Now, if you were the doctor who would you rather take care of? Which person's diagnosis seems clearer to you? Which patient do you think will be more likely to get the right tests, diagnosis, and treatments the first time? How might that affect your health — or your wealth?

The patient in the second example is more focused and has given his symptoms some thought. The doctor hasn't needed to interrupt the patient or ask questions because the information being given is important. The first patient, however, only seemed to focus on the fact that he was tired and had little else to offer. Since his history was less helpful, there is a better chance that more tests will be done, perhaps even unnecessarily.

Wise patients appear to know instinctively what to say and ask. They prepare before their visit to get the most out of it. To ensure that the doctor gets all of the information he needs, the wise patient provides him with a detailed medical history.

First, Set the Agenda

Before you go into the doctor's office, *decide what you want to discuss with your doctor by setting an agenda for the visit.* Doctors appreciate this greatly. It helps them figure out how much time to devote to each problem. Is the patient in for a physical and to receive preventive care and tests? Does the patient have a new problem that needs a medical evaluation, or an ongoing problem that requires follow-up or further treatment?

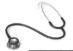 **Real-Life Example**

> A twenty-year-old woman saw me once for breast pain. After a thorough history and examination, I determined that her pain was related to her monthly periods, was nothing serious, and fairly common. She appeared to leave the appointment satisfied, so naturally I was puzzled when she returned to my office a couple of months later for the same problem.
>
> After determining again that it was nothing serious, before I finished, I asked her what she was worried about. She was concerned about breast cancer. Since I had never explicitly told her she didn't have cancer, she was still worried. Breast cancer was her concern and that was her agenda. From a medical perspective, breast cancer in a twenty-year-old is rare, but for her the fear was real. Based on her examination, I reassured her she had nothing to worry about and encouraged her to see me if any changes occurred. She was relieved.

Bringing up the most important issue at the end of the visit, particularly as you are about to leave the doctor's office, is extremely frustrating for the physician. You might also shortchange yourself by not having enough time to adequately explain your concerns or questions. If you want to talk about four concerns, tell your doctor at the beginning of the visit that you want to talk about four items and list them, without going into too much detail at first. Be sure to indicate which one is the most important to you. This will help the doctor enormously.

Example: Agenda of a Wise Patient

> **Doctor:** What brings you in today?
>
> **Patient:** Well, Doctor, I want to talk about four things today. First, I've been feeling tired. Second, I have this nagging ankle pain. Third, this spot on my back. And finally, these headaches.

According to one study, family physicians spent about seventeen minutes per patient visit and internists about nineteen and a half minutes.[42] In that short time, patients and doctors need to cover everything from patient concerns, a physical examination, and a discussion of appropriate tests, medications, and follow up.

If at all possible, I recommend tackling no more than four concerns in your office visit, especially if the four are new problems never before evaluated by your doctor. The goal is not to cram in as many problems as possible in a visit, but rather to get the most out of the visit by getting an accurate diagnosis and treatment plan. The aim is quality, not quantity.

Be sure you know which problem is most important to you in case your doctor feels like he can't cover everything. A good doctor will not only pick the problem that is most important (i.e. the one that's potentially life threatening), but also will realize that it is far better for your health to discuss a few issues in depth rather than too many items superficially. So,

The goal is not to cram in as many problems as possible in a visit, but rather to get the most out of the visit by getting an accurate diagnosis and treatment plan. The aim is quality, not quantity.

write up a list of problems and questions you wish to discuss and make the number manageable.

Next, Tackle Each Issue: When, What, Where, and Why

Once you have set the agenda for the visit, it's time to discuss each problem in detail and avoid being interrupted too quickly by your doctor. Ask him which problem he wants to tackle first. Alternatively, you can just begin by talking about each problem in depth.

Always tell your problem the same way you might tell a story. Give it a beginning, a middle, and an end. It is, after all, *your* story about your symptoms and problems, and it is much easier for your doctor to follow the sequence of events this way. Start in chronological order. While this may seem obvious, you'd be surprised how many patients don't start at the beginning. They talk about their symptoms in no particular order and blurt out whatever thoughts enter their heads.

To help you organize your thoughts, use the Four Ws — the when, what, where, and why. The Four Ws help enhance your story to make sure that important details aren't overlooked. Your doctor may ask you to clarify or expand on details if you forget them. Organizing your thoughts logically using the Four Ws brings a level of sophistication and detail to the office visit that decreases the likelihood that you will be interrupted or that the doctor won't get the information he needs.

First year medical students use a similar format to elicit a comprehensive history from patients. Although the format may seem complicated at first, with practice not only will you start thinking about your problems in this way, you may also begin to think and express yourself like a doctor! Start with the when, the what, and the where.

When:

> ➤ When did you first notice the problem? Describe how the problem has changed over time.

➤ When does it seem to occur?

➤ When was the last time you had the problem?

What:

➤ What activities, treatments, or behaviors seem to make the problem better, worse, or no different (this can include home therapies like taking over-the-counter medications, applying heat or ice, eating or not eating, going to the bathroom, movement, activity or lack of, etc., depending on the problem).

➤ What does the problem feel like? How would you describe the pain (i.e. sharp, dull, burning, gnawing, pressure-like, tight, achy, constant, increasing, comes and goes).

➤ What other problems or symptoms have you noticed?

Where:

➤ Where did the problem start? Did it move over time, and if so, where?

➤ Does the pain or condition move anywhere else in the body?

Finally, end with the why. The why is the reason you are at the doctor's office. While you don't have to provide this information, as it may be completely obvious, doctors may ask when it isn't clear why. Reasons are personal and quite varied.

Why:

➤ I want to make sure it isn't anything serious, like cancer or a heart attack.

➤ I wanted to make sure I don't need to take antibiotics, change my behavior, or forego my vacation.

➤ The problem is interfering with my lifestyle.

➤ My wife/husband/family member is worried about my problem.

The examples below illustrate how vital a good personal history is, and how helpful the four Ws can be for delivering a comprehensive history.

 Examples of Personal Histories Using the Four Ws

Patient: I have this rash. It started about three days ago on the arm (when and where). It's not really itchy (what — other symptoms), and I haven't tried anything for it (what — better/worse). I feel well otherwise. But I wanted to make sure it wasn't serious (why).

OR

Patient: I think I'm depressed. I think I first noticed it about three months ago when I started my new job (when). I've been more stressed lately and eating more. I've been crying more, been more irritable, and not feeling like doing anything (what — associated symptoms). It used to help if I exercised, but now even that doesn't help. I can't stay asleep. I keep waking in the early morning tossing and turning. I tried some over-the-counter medication for sleep which didn't help (what — better/worse). I've never been diagnosed with depression before (when). I don't know what to do (why).

OR

Patient: I think I have a sinus infection. It started about two weeks ago (when) with a head cold (what — other symptoms). It began with a sore throat, runny nose, muscle aches all over, and I just wasn't feeling well (what and where). I took some over-the-counter cold medications which seemed to help, as did warm showers (what — better/worse). I didn't have any fever. I did have a little cough (what — other symptoms). Over the past few days, my sinuses have been hurting and now I have a fever and am blowing greenish stuff from my nose (when — how symptoms changed over time). I'm going on a trip to Europe in the next few days and want to see if I need any antibiotics or if this will get better on its own (why).

OR

Patient: I wanted to talk about my back pain. Over the past week (when) I've been having low back pain (what) that comes and goes, lasting for about twenty minutes (when). The pain is really intense and feels like someone is stabbing me with a knife (what). I tried some Tylenol, but really, nothing makes it better or worse (what — better/worse). It seems to come on without any warning (when). The pain is mostly on the right side (where) and I couldn't sleep last night. Lying down, sitting, or standing makes no difference (what — better/ worse). I haven't had any pain in the legs. I haven't had any problems with my urine or problems going to the bathroom. No fever, nausea, vomiting, or diarrhea (what — other symptoms). I've never had this before (when — last time had problem). I'm not sure what it is and what to do (why).

Once you finish describing your first problem, move on to the others using a similar format. Although it does take some time to think about how to fill in the details about a particular issue, the payoff is that your doctor will have plenty of information to work with. This will increase the chance of him providing you with the right diagnosis and treatment.

Avoid the urge to diagnose yourself and say things like "I have the flu." Although it seems like convenient shorthand, doctors are very specific with terminology and what you mean could be completely different than what a doctor understands the term to mean. Going to medical school is like immersing yourself in a foreign country. In four years medical students learn an entirely different culture, language, and perspective on the world. Their new vocabulary provides them the precision, understanding, and tools to communicate with their peers. Perhaps it isn't surprising that many doctors have forgotten how to speak normally!

By the way, the flu is an illness that causes a sudden onset of headache, high fever, cough that does not produce phlegm, and sore throat. It typically resolves within one week.[43] Patients' interpretation of the flu usually varies from symptoms consistent with food poisoning (nausea, vomiting, and diarrhea), a kidney infection (fever, back pain, vomiting), to pneumonia. Obviously, treatment for each of these conditions is quite different.

Instead of self diagnosing, talk about your symptoms. This doesn't mean you can't ask questions like, "Do you think I have a pinched disc in my back?" or "Do you think I have pneumonia?" or say things like, "These symptoms remind me of the time I had pneumonia." If you have had the problem in the past, go ahead and tell your doctor. Many times these comments are very helpful.

Putting It All Together

So you provided an excellent history and hopefully weren't interrupted too often. As you started to provide details, your doctor was already pondering the possible diagnoses. If you complained of back pain which got worse with movement, got better with a warm towel or massage, and was painful to the touch, then he is likely to conclude the culprit was a muscle pull or strain.

If the back pain instead was accompanied by fever and vomiting, and you have a history of bladder infections, then the most likely diagnosis is a kidney infection. If you described your pain as gradually becoming more severe, associated with weight loss, not better with rest or inactivity, and starting to keep you awake at night, the doctor might entertain a more worrisome diagnosis like cancer.

If none of these potential diagnoses fits your complaints and initial observations, your doctor may ask additional questions to determine whether other diagnoses like a pinched nerve, a kidney stone, or shingles (a skin condition also known as herpes zoster) could be the source of the pain.

Wise patients know that getting an accurate diagnosis requires that their doctors have all the information they need. Describing your problems in a concise format, using the four Ws, means you may require fewer visits and thus save time and money.

KNOW YOURSELF — YOUR PERSONAL MEDICAL HISTORY

> "Knowing your family's history can save your life."
> — U.S. Surgeon General Richard Carmona (November 2004)

Although knowing how to present yourself efficiently and effectively is a great way to start getting the most out of your health care, you also need to know about your personal medical history to stay healthy. Surprisingly, many patients often do not know their medical history or family medical history. Others are apathetic because they feel that certain diseases are inevitable, are part of the family history, or are a normal part of aging.

Understanding your personal medical history may cause you to consider interventions that could alter your future health and outcome, improve your quality of life, and decrease your chances of premature death.

Understanding your personal medical history may cause you to consider interventions that could alter your future health and outcome, improve your quality of life, and decrease your chances of premature death. To know yourself well and increase your chances of staying healthy, focus on these four important areas: your medical/surgical history, family medical history, medications/allergies, and, finally, social history.

Past Medical/Surgical History

Your past medical/surgical history simply details any situations or medical conditions that might be important for your doctor to know. Think about situations which required repeated treatments or office visits.

Start chronologically with your childhood. Did you have a serious illness, require hospitalization, or have an operation? If so, do you have more details about the diagnosis and treatment? Are you still having any problems? Do you have a history of surgery your doctor should know about? How about abdominal surgery? Do you have any medical problems that require you take medications daily? When were you first diagnosed and what was the illness? Have you ever had cancer? Is there any other medical information you think your doctor should know?

A physician will approach a patient complaining of abdominal pain very differently depending on whether the patient has a) had gallbladder and/or appendix surgery; b) a history of colon cancer; or c) no surgical history at all. In the first instance, the gallbladder or appendix couldn't be the cause of the pain, since one or both were removed. In the second instance, the doctor might be concerned that the colon cancer has returned. And in the third instance, all of the above diagnoses are possible.

Medications and Allergies

Consider the next section, medications/allergies. Are you currently taking medications, including prescribed drugs, over-the-counter remedies, herbal remedies, or dietary supplements on a regular basis? What is the actual name of the medication and the dosage? How often do you take it? What do you take it for? Have you taken other medications in the past for the same problem? Do you remember why you switched medications? (Often, patients will switch medication brands because the previous medication was not helpful, had too many side effects, or the insurance company no longer provided coverage for the pill.) Obviously, if a medication failed to be effective in the past, it will be wise to avoid it in the future. Other times, medications can cause problems either during or after treatment. Don't be embarrassed or afraid to tell your doctor the reason you stopped a medication was because it was too expensive. Physicians are often busy and don't realize the financial cost of the treatments they prescribe. It's better to be honest.

Astute patients know it is their responsibility to keep track of what medications they are taking, how often they are taking them, and the reasons for taking them. By knowing what you are taking and ensuring that your doctor also knows, you decrease the chance that he will write a new prescription that interferes with your current medication.

Although some patients may feel it is the doctor's responsibility to check the medication list for accuracy and know what his patient is

> *Although some patients may feel it is the doctor's responsibility to check the medication list for accuracy and know what his patient is taking, ultimately it is the individual's health at stake, not the doctor's.*

taking, ultimately it is the individual's health at stake, not the doctor's. Only patients will know what they are taking and how often. Doctors often write prescriptions that patients either don't fill or don't take as directed because they're concerned about side effects, don't believe they need treatment, or can't afford the medication. As a result, the doctor's medical chart will not match the patient's.

If individuals don't know *why* they are taking something, it is the responsibility of the doctor to tell them. He should educate a patient when asked. So if you don't know, or are unsure, ask. Don't be embarrassed. It happens often. I would rather have a patient ask me at each visit than have someone unsure and scared about their treatment.

Once you've told your doctor all the medications you're taking, consider allergies. Have you ever experienced any side effects or allergies from medications? Allergies or sensitivities to food? If so, which ones? And more importantly, what were your symptoms?

For many patients, some antibiotics can cause stomach upset, nausea, loose stools, or a rash. These symptoms are often not an actual *allergy*, but a medication side effect. True allergies can include certain types of rashes, difficulty breathing, and hives, among others.

Many patients with medication side effects are erroneously labeled with medication allergies. Consequently, patients might be prescribed more expensive medications, which may not be any more effective. Talk to your doctor about your symptoms so that he can determine the medication side effects from allergies.

Family History

Your family medical history can also impact your health, so it's important to share it with your doctor. Focus first on your immediate family, your parents and siblings. Since they are the most genetically related to you, knowing and understanding the illnesses that affected them can help you and your doctor take action to minimize the likelihood that you will develop the same problems.

Despite what many people think, diabetes and many other illnesses are not necessarily a normal consequence of aging.

Initiating early intervention and treatment can improve your quality of life and decrease your risk of complications. Does anyone in your immediate family have diabetes? A history of heart disease or heart attacks? Cancer? Strokes? High blood pressure? If so, at what age were they diagnosed? Did they have any complications from the illness? Are there any other illnesses that occur in your family?

For example, patients with a family history of diabetes would know that they could prevent or delay the onset of diabetes with exercise, diet changes, and maintaining a healthy weight. They could partner with their doctor and have an annual blood sugar test to monitor their progress as well as detect the illness at its earliest stages. Research has shown that patients who adopt exercise and healthy dietary habits decrease their risk of developing the disease far better than if they started taking prescription medication to prevent diabetes.

Despite what many people think, diabetes and many other illnesses are not necessarily a normal consequence of aging. Some people age better than others; many of my older patients do not have diabetes, heart disease, or osteoporosis. Still, patients surprise me when they reply that no one in the family has medical problems. When pushed they answer, "Just the usual, Doc. Diabetes, heart attacks, and high blood pressure. Nothing serious."

Social History

Finally, focus on you and everything else about you. Understanding you as an individual gives your doctor some insights into how your lifestyle can impact your health. Who are you? What makes you different from other patients? What is your occupation? What kind of work do you do and what does that involve? Who lives with you at home? Do you smoke? Do you drink alcohol? Do you have any history of recent or past drug use? Are you sexually active? Do you do any regular exercise or physical activity? All of this information is detailed in what's called the social history.

Your behaviors, lifestyle, and environment can help determine your risk of developing future medical problems. If your family has a history of early heart disease, your smoking habit would dramatically increase your risk of developing early heart disease yourself. If, on the other hand, you exercised regularly, quit smoking, lowered your cholesterol, and took an aspirin daily, you would decrease your risk and improve your chances of achieving good health.

While we have portrayed the medical history, family history, and social history as potential liabilities or problems that could prevent you from obtaining good health, understanding them provides an opportunity for you to do better. Do you walk or exercise regularly? Have you had the appropriate tests for cholesterol and the cancer screenings that are recommended for your age and gender? Have you quit smoking or decreased your alcohol consumption? (Congratulations if you have — those are hard habits to beat.) Are you up to date on your vaccinations? Do you protect yourself by wearing seat belts, helmets, and other protective gear when needed? Are you at a healthy weight? While you cannot control your family history or your situation, you can change your current habits, and therefore improve your chances of maintaining good health.

Before you see your physician, think about your own personal medical history, your family medical history, medications and allergies, and your social history. Type this information on a sheet of paper and give it to your physician to add to your medical chart. Update it periodically.

Following is an example.

Joe Smith   **Date of Birth 1/21/1962**

Last updated 1/7/2007
Past Medical History
High blood pressure — diagnosed 2002
Hayfever
Heartburn

Past Surgical History
Appendectomy at age 18

Family History
Mother — high blood pressure at age 55
Father — diabetes at age 68; prostate cancer at age 75
Both parents alive and well
No family history of heart disease or stroke

Medications
Hydrochlorothiazide 25 mg per day for high blood pressure
Claritin (loratadine) 10 mg per day as needed for allergies
Pepcid (famotidine) 20 mg 2 times per day as needed for
     heartburn

Allergies
Penicillin caused a rash. No hives or breathing difficulties.

Social History
Quit smoking 3 years ago. Smoked 1 pack per day for 20 years.
Do not drink alcohol. Married with 2 children ages 10 and 12.
Work as a computer programmer. Get a flu vaccine annually.

Make your own medical history form by using the template below.

Name:_____

Date of Birth: _____ / _____ / _____

Last Updated: _____ / _____ / _____

Past Medical History (list any problems that you know about, even if you don't need prescription medication): _____

_____

_____

_____

Past Surgical History (list any surgeries and indicate your age when they occurred):

_____

_____

Family History (include problems like high blood pressure, diabetes, cancer, heart disease, and emphysema. Indicate the age when the illness was first diagnosed.):

Mother _____

Father _____

Siblings_____

_____

_____

Medications (list the name, dosage, how often you are taking it, and the reason):

_____

_____

_____

_____

Allergies (indicate medication and the specific symptoms they caused — i.e. rash, hives, nausea, or diarrhea): _____

_____

_____

_____

Social History (include whether you smoke or drink, your marital/relationship status, and occupation): _____

_____

_____

_____

_____

MAKE EVERY OFFICE VISIT COUNT

Now that you know how to present yourself effectively and have thoroughly reviewed your medical history, you still need to make every office visit count.

Always be frank and up front with your doctor. While there are certain facts and behaviors some patients would never admit to even their own significant others or parents, knowledgeable patients know that withholding any information could complicate things. Don't be embarrassed.

Doctors learn in medical school that people are very different in their lifestyles, habits, and concerns. Therefore, there are no silly questions. Ask the questions, tell the doctor your concerns, and be honest. Accurate diagnoses and treatments depend on your honesty and accuracy. *Doctors are trained to be nonjudgmental.* If you use illicit drugs, are underage and drink, or do not want to take medication for your problem, it is okay to discuss these issues with your doctor. If you forgot to take your medications correctly or as prescribed, be honest. If you take a friend's or family member's prescription medication — which is never a good idea — you need to let the doctor know. Otherwise he might prescribe a medication that interferes with it or give you the same treatment.

If you feel that you can't have an honest discussion with your doctor or are uncomfortable with him, you may want to consider finding a new physician. The most vital part of a doctor-patient relationship is the element of trust.

If you feel that you can't have an honest discussion with your doctor or are uncomfortable with him, you may want to consider finding a new physician. The most vital part of a doctor-patient relationship is the element of trust.

Also, be respectful and courteous to physicians and their office staff. Turn off your cell phone, Blackberry, or pager before you enter the exam room so you and your doctor can focus entirely on your visit. Always address your doctor by his professional name, unless directed otherwise. Cancel appointments you are unable to make as some offices will charge patients who don't show up (sometimes a small fee, sometimes the full cost of the visit). Other medical groups terminate or see only on a walk-in basis patients who chronically miss appointments.[44]

A 1996 study at the Mayo Clinic showed that patients remember less than half of what physicians tell them during office visits.

In today's society, where being polite appears to be the exception rather than the rule, wise patients know that being considerate makes a difference. You can get your concerns and points across and still be respectful. Physicians and staff, like patients, get sick, have bad days, and have family problems too. Wise patients realize that friendliness, a smile, and common sense can go a long way to making the patient-doctor relationship a good one.

Finally, the most important point of the entire visit is to remember what happened. What did you and your doctor talk about? What was the diagnosis? What was the treatment plan? What did you decide to do? When do you need to come back? A 1996 study at the Mayo Clinic showed that patients remember less than half of what physicians tell them during office visits.[45] Of nearly 600 patients who were asked to recall what diagnoses physicians had discussed with them, 54 percent could not remember the major problems. Of patients whose doctors had discussed with them the risk factors for heart disease, 68 percent did not recall any discussion about tobacco use, 62 percent did not remember hypertension (high blood pressure), and 73 percent did not recall obesity.

D.A.T.E.

When leaving the appointment, wise patients will do well to remember the acronym D.A.T.E. By remembering the D.A.T.E., the patient knows what he or she needs to do to get better or find out what is wrong.

D. Did you understand and remember the (D)iagnosis? If not, ask the doctor to write it down. Get the actual medical terminology rather than layman's wording. Bring your own paper and pen if you have to, particularly if this is not a typical visit for something relatively benign like a cold. *The diagnosis is critical.* When my brother was evaluated for a lump on his shoulder, he was told only that he had a growth that needed to be operated on. Only after he called me and I pressed him for the actual diagnosis and exact medical terminology did we realize that his lump was a rare muscle cancer, a sarcoma. I encouraged him to get care at a specialized medical center where he had a chance for cure through a very precise and specific surgery. Had he stayed with his other doctor, he had a 50 percent chance that the cancer would come back. His doctor admitted to my brother that he honestly didn't know what the lump was, but that it needed to come out.

Never ever accept the phrase, "we'll only contact you if the results are bad."

Knowing the exact diagnosis made it possible for my brother to choose a surgical specialist who would perform one surgery that would cure him versus having a general surgeon do a simple removal and having a good chance the tumor would come back.

A. Does your doctor require or recommend any (A)dditional testing, x-rays, or procedures? Is additional input from other doctors, usually specialists, important? Do you need a referral? Does the doctor need your medical records from other doctors' offices or hospitals?

If additional testing is needed, remember to always make sure that your doctor has seen the results. Never ever accept the phrase, "we'll only contact you if the results are bad." What if your doctor never sees the results because of misfiled paperwork or a laboratory mix-up? What if your doctor and/or his office never got the results and never contacted you? You were told not to worry unless someone called. So who pays the ultimate price for this oversight? You do.

I tell my patients, *no news means no news.* The news could be good or bad, and you won't know unless you are contacted with the results. So, if any additional testing is needed, you should always expect to get the results. They can be communicated to you through a simple letter, postcard, or phone call from the office staff. Call your doctor if you don't hear from him in a reasonable amount of time. It is always better to double check and be safe than sorry.

T. Is it clear to you what the (T)reatment plan is? Are you starting medications or changing dosages? Do you need to see a physical therapist to treat your knee pain? Do you need to attend any preventive health classes? Do you need to exercise more? What are the treatment goals and plans?

E. Finally, when should you return for further (E)xaminations or (E)valuations? Do you return in a few days, weeks, months, or a year for a follow-up visit? Who makes the appointment? What signs or symptoms should you look out for which would indicate that you need to be seen sooner?

Remember, the D.A.T.E. you had with your doctor, and the hard work you put into achieving a high-quality visit will pay off.

Establish Visit

For a variety of reasons, we need to switch physicians periodically. Employers switch health insurance plans almost as often as physicians join and leave them. Or we might change jobs and our new employer's plan differs from our previous one. A new insurance plan usually means choosing a new physician. Sometimes, people change doctors because they no longer feel comfortable with their physician, or because their previous doctor retired or left the community. If you aren't happy with your doctor's care, let him know before you switch. After discussing your concerns with him, you may decide to stay.

Do yourself a favor: get your medical records, make a copy for yourself, and bring the other copy to your new physician.

When meeting a new doctor, the most important visit is the *establish visit*. This refers to the first visit the patient has with his new doctor, and is particularly vital for patients with multiple chronic medical problems or multiple prescription medications. (I would define a chronic medical problem as a condition that requires a patient take medication daily to stay healthy. Conditions that would fit this category include asthma, diabetes, high blood pressure, heart disease, high cholesterol, emphysema, and congestive heart failure, among others.)

Seeing your doctor when you feel well has a couple of benefits. First, it shows your physician that you are new to his practice. And second, it shows your doctor that you care enough about your health to make a routine visit to meet him and review any chronic medical problems that require continued monitoring and treatment.

Before making your first appointment, get your medical records from your previous doctor. You can talk to the receptionist or office staff about how to get those records. You will either need to sign paperwork or mail a letter giving your old doctor permission to send your confidential medical information to your new doctor. Even if you are charged to copy your records, the cost is worth it. Without your old records for reference, your new doctor may repeat expensive tests or procedures that were already performed. Not only will you need to go through the inconvenience of repeating the same test, but you will also be stuck with additional out-of-pocket costs. Do yourself a favor: get your medical records, make a copy for yourself, and bring the other copy to your new physician.

If you are also enrolled in a new health insurance plan, you may discover that some of your medications are no longer covered. Seeing your doctor when you are well is a good time to consider changing to alternative medications which *are* covered. And should you have any side effects or problems, they will be readily apparent to you and your physician.

The goal of the establish visit is to avoid a stressful new patient visit in which an individual with chronic medical problems and multiple medications comes in for an urgent appointment with a doctor who knows nothing about the patient. With an establish visit, you can ensure that you've met your doctor — and that your doctor knows your history — before things become urgent.

The urgent visit is often terribly confusing and difficult for both doctor and patient. Which patient would you rather be? The one who comes in with an acute problem but has met his new doctor, who knows his medical history already? Or the one who comes in with an urgent problem and meets a new doctor who has no medical information about his patient? Which patient will have the better outcome?

The establish visit also helps you decide if this doctor and his style are right for you. When you are feeling well, it's easier to familiarize yourself with the office and staff and evaluate your physician. If you are not comfortable with the practice, you can then work on changing doctors until you find one you do like. If you wait until the urgent appointment to address all of your problems, you don't have much choice about whether you like your new physician's practice and ideology — you just need to see a doctor!

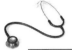 **Real-Life Example**

A few years ago, I took my in-laws to see a new doctor for an establish visit. My father-in-law, who was chronically ill with many aliments, rarely saw doctors, but he had recently gotten health insurance, so it seemed like an opportune time for him to have an establish visit. My wife, who is a doctor, summarized her father's medical history and listed his medications in a one-page letter.

The letter helped tremendously. My father-in-law's new physician introduced himself and quickly looked over the letter and my father-in-law's medical history. The doctor asked him how he was feeling and some other specific questions. At the end of the visit, his doctor had a good sense of what needed to be done to continue to care for him. My father-in-law was now effectively "plugged in" to the new insurance plan's system. Prescription medications were refilled, blood tests were drawn, and referrals to specialists were completed. We were all confident that should he require future care, the doctors would have the necessary information to keep him healthy.

As I returned home after dropping off my in-laws I wondered, *why don't other people do that for themselves?* Of the many patients I see, only a handful of those with chronic medical problems present themselves with a one-page medical summary, and even fewer come in for an establish visit before a crisis happens.

My advice is to take it upon yourself, when you are new to a doctor, to make an appointment for an establish visit.

A Second Opinion Visit

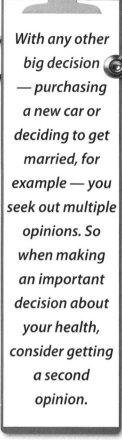

With any other big decision — purchasing a new car or deciding to get married, for example — you seek out multiple opinions. So when making an important decision about your health, consider getting a second opinion.

Doctors are sometimes patients and aren't afraid to ask for a second opinion. You shouldn't be either. With any other big decision — purchasing a new car or deciding to get married, for example — you seek out multiple opinions. So when making an important decision about your health, consider getting a second opinion. Good doctors realize that sometimes patients need to discuss their conditions with another doctor or get two opinions before they can move on. These opinions may or may not be the same.

Getting a second opinion can be initiated by the patient, the patient's family, the patient's physician, or, sometimes, by the insurance company. It can be as simple as a patient saying to his or her doctor, "It would help me make a decision regarding the care you're suggesting if I had a second opinion. Can you arrange it for me?" Alternatively, the physician or the insurance company might recommend a patient seek a second opinion. You shouldn't worry that your doctor might be offended by the question. Physicians who are confident about their abilities and diagnoses understand. Many, if given the same circumstance as a patient, would demand a second opinion.

For a patient diagnosed with a rare illness, having a second opinion can confirm or refute the original diagnosis. Obviously, this could have enormous consequences on long term prognosis and treatment options. Other patients might seek out doctors who can offer alternative kinds of treatments or other perspectives. Second opinions can confirm previous doctors' recommendations or provide a new perspective on the same problem. In any of these cases, it's important to understand why you are having a second opinion and to come prepared to the visit.

Why you are going for a second opinion? Why do you want to go? What do you hope to learn from the visit? How will a second opinion change what you already know?

Suppose you were recently diagnosed with a rare kidney disease. You and your doctor arrange a second opinion with a specialist at a university hospital. You might ask the doctor the following questions:

➤ Is the initial diagnosis the correct diagnosis?

➤ If not, then what is the correct diagnosis? How does this change the treatment and prognosis?

➤ If the diagnosis is correct, is the treatment that was recommended by the previous doctor appropriate and reasonable?

➤ Does the previous doctor have adequate experience in treatment of this condition, or would the treatment be better if performed by the university hospital staff?

➤ Is there an alternative treatment available?

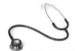 **Real-Life Example**

> Earlier I wrote about my brother, Dennis, who developed a hard lump on his shoulder that was initially evaluated by his dermatologist. The doctor wasn't sure what the lump was, and referred him to a surgeon for a biopsy. The biopsy was performed in the office under local anesthesia. When the results came back, my parents and Dennis were not told explicitly that the condition was in fact a rare muscle cancer. The surgeon simply recommended that the lump be removed under general

anesthesia in the operating room. Although both the referring dermatologist and the surgeon knew of the condition, neither had experience with the disease.

A week before his scheduled surgery we discovered the biopsy's true diagnosis. And when we reviewed his medical records, we discovered that the original pathologist (a specialist who interprets tissue samples and biopsies) had had his entire department review the biopsy sample to confirm his findings. They all agreed on the diagnosis: a rare cancer with a very high recurrence rate of about 50 percent.

Because the cancer was rare, and because both of my brother's doctors had not had any personal experience with the illness, we insisted that Dennis cancel his surgery and seek a second opinion from a musculoskeletal oncologist, an orthopedic surgeon with additional fellowship training on cancer of the muscles and bones. We discovered that only two physicians in the state had the training and the experience to treat his cancer.

Dennis and my parents met his new doctor at the university hospital. His case was reevaluated by the university pathologists, who agreed with the original diagnosis. His doctor recommended a pre-operative MRI to assess the tumor size. The MRI, they advised, would also help in planning the surgical approach and technique to minimize recurrence. In the specialist's experience, and with his methodology, there was a 95 percent cure rate — far better than the 50 percent recurrence rate the other procedure would have ensured.

Ultimately, Dennis chose to have the university hospital surgical team remove the tumor since they had years of experience. Today, he is doing well, living cancer-free. While we will never know if getting a second opinion truly changed his outcome, I am convinced that it did. The rare cancer he had required treatment by a surgeon with the unique experience and expertise. Anything less would have increased his risk of recurrence, future surgeries, or worse.

Make the most of your second opinion visit by coming prepared. Ideally, if your doctor is requesting a second opinion, he has already sent a letter of introduction about your case or called the consulting physician to provide some background information. But this won't always happen.

To ensure that the consulting physician has the information he needs, send all of your relevant medical records, lab tests, and x-ray reports to the office before your appointment. The more information the consulting doctor has, the better he can render an accurate opinion and diagnosis. Finally, if you are able to get a copy for yourself, do. It never hurts to set up a file for yourself. Make an extra copy and bring it to your visit.

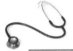 **Real Life Example**

When my wife, Jocelyn, trained as an oncology fellow at a large university medical center, she often provided a second opinion for many cancer patients. The hospital received referrals from community oncologists who wanted help in treating patients who had rare cancers, unclear diagnoses, complications with cancer treatment, or who had not benefited from standard chemotherapy treatment.

The oncologists she worked with cared for patients with the toughest cases as well as the most unusual. Collectively, they had much more experience with treatment of rare cancer types than an individual doctor would get over an entire career. They treated patients with new experimental chemotherapy regimens.

While they had plenty to offer, treatment could not begin until the university medical staff had reviewed patients' medical records and test results from their previous or referring doctors. Only by reviewing the old medical records, copies of old x-rays, pathology reports, or lab tests, could they establish accurate diagnoses and develop treatment plans. Without having the actual biopsy slides, her colleagues in pathology could not confirm or refute any diagnosis. New chemotherapy or radiation treatments could not be initiated until they knew what treatment options were tried in the past. Patient care was often delayed.

This scenario happens too often everywhere. It frustrated my wife to see referred patients without any medical records or other critical information. Until the old medical records arrived and were thoroughly reviewed, initiating treatment would need to wait.

The lesson is to call ahead. Find out what your second opinion physician needs. Get your medical records.

INFORMED CONSENT: IS IT OKAY WITH YOU?

In the past, the doctor-patient relationship was dominated by the physician. It was believed that patients did not have adequate knowledge or the ability to truly understand the risks and benefits of medical treatments or procedures since the physicians had all the training and education. Whatever the doctor felt was in the best interest of the patient, regardless of what the patient thought, would be done. It was a very paternalistic relationship.

Over time, the doctor-patient relationship has evolved to one of shared responsibility.

Over time, the doctor-patient relationship has evolved to one of shared responsibility. Although patients generally do not have the expertise or depth of medical knowledge that clinicians do, the idea behind *informed consent* is that when patients are given adequate information that is appropriate to their level of understanding, they can make decisions that are more consistent with their needs. While the decision may not be what the physician recommends, as long as the patient fully understands the benefits, risks, and alternatives to having a treatment or procedure done, the decision he makes is fine. (This assumes, of course, that the patient can make decisions, i.e. does not suffer from dementia and is not a danger to himself or others.)

These days, one of the roles of a physician is to provide information and guidance for individuals to make their own medical decisions. To ensure that patients have adequate information to give informed consent, a physician is supposed to provide the patient with all the information he needs. This can be implicit, something that occurs over the course of an office visit, or can be more explicit and detailed, with a formal discussion of treatment options, as well as paperwork.

In order for a patient to give informed consent, the physician needs to answer the following questions:

➤ What are the benefits of having a particular treatment or procedure done?

➤ What are the risks or complications of the treatment or procedure?

➤ What are the alternative treatment options or procedures?

The following scenario illustrates informed consent: a doctor provides a woman with all her options for dealing with a lump in her breast. In this way she can make an informed decision about diagnosis and treatment. The physician recommends a breast biopsy to be performed in the operating room.

> **Doctor:** The reason we will be doing a breast biopsy is to find out if the lump is something serious, like cancer. The benefit of doing the procedure is finding out exactly what the breast lump is — it could be benign or malignant.
>
> The risks of the biopsy are similar to those of any surgical procedure. These can include infection, bleeding, scarring, risks related to anesthesia (including death), and the need to have additional surgery in the future, among others. Overall, however, the risks are low, with the most common being infection, bleeding, or the need for additional surgery.
>
> The alternative option is to have a stereotactic biopsy done, in which a computer aided by a mammogram can do multiple biopsies of the lump using a needle. This procedure has fewer complications than surgery, but it isn't

perfect. The biopsies may miss the lump, which would mean later surgery to determine whether the mass is serious. If the biopsies show cancer, surgery would still be required to remove the lump.

Another alternative would be to do nothing and observe the lump and see if it grows over the next few months. I do not recommend this option, as the potential for the lump to be something serious is much higher than the chance that it's benign.

Understandably, despite informed consent, some patients don't wish to make a decision and prefer that the physicians do instead. As long as the doctor has provided a patient with the opportunity to be informed, it's appropriate for the doctor to make the decision. At any time, patients can give up or take back more responsibility of the shared decision making. The most important thing is that they be given the opportunity to be informed of the benefits, risks, and alternatives to having any treatment or procedure performed.

DON'T SEE YOUR DOCTOR

Despite everything we've discussed, it's obvious that you can cut your health care costs by *not* seeing your doctor. Wise patients, therefore, will choose when to see their doctor and when not to.

What should you consider an unnecessary visit? Naturally, simple coughs and colds in otherwise healthy adults probably don't need the care of a doctor; they require time, rest, and patience. But how do you know something is a simple cough or cold? While you might ask yourself, *if I didn't have insurance, would I go see a doctor?* This probably isn't the best way of determining when to go.

A useful resource is www.familydoctor.org, from the American Academy of Family Physicians. This website has flowsheets of symptoms, and can guide you to determining whether a medical evaluation is needed (look under the Health Tools section). Alternatively, purchasing a good home medical reference book is just as valuable, and wise patients will have such a book on their bookshelves.

After referring to these reference guides, if you *do* think you need care, see if it can be handled over the telephone. Use some common sense. For example, women who are otherwise healthy who find they have an uncomplicated bladder infection can often be treated with antibiotics and don't need to visit the doctor. There are other situations where a phone call would suffice as well. The only way to find out is to call the office or your insurance company, which may have a twenty-four-hour advice line, and inquire about your symptoms. If they recommend you go to the doctor, you should go. And if they recommend a simple prescription but you still feel uncomfortable and would rather see your doctor in person, do it. It is ultimately your decision and your health.

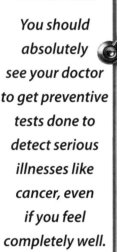

You should absolutely see your doctor to get preventive tests done to detect serious illnesses like cancer, even if you feel completely well.

You should absolutely see your doctor to get preventive tests done to detect serious illnesses like cancer, even if you feel completely well. Cancer caught early increases the chance of cure and decreases the likelihood that you will need expensive chemotherapies or extensive surgeries and procedures. Despite fancier technology and treatment options, most physicians agree that prevention and early intervention is the most successful way to keep people healthy and living longer. Refer to the next section to see what tests you should definitely ask your physician for in order to stay healthy.

TAKE-HOME POINTS

✓ *Maximize your office visit and provide the perfect history.* Be an effective storyteller. Set the agenda and focus on the what, where, when, and why for each issue. Give your physician the information he needs to accurately diagnose you. A good history may decrease the need for additional testing.

✓ *Know yourself.* Review your medical history, surgical history, medications you are taking, allergies, family medical history, and social history.

✓ *Make every office visit count.* Use common sense. Be courteous. Be honest.

✓ *When you leave an office visit, be sure you have made a D.A.T.E. with your doctor.* You know your (D)iagnosis; any necessary (A)dditional tests or procedures; the (T)reatment for the problem; and when you need future (E)xaminations or (E)valuations.

✓ *Remember that no news means no news.* If you get any testing done, always expect to get the results. If you aren't notified, call your doctor. Better to be safe than sorry.

✓ *Consider establishing a visit with your new physician before you have any acute or urgent problems.* This is important for patients with chronic illnesses or those who take many prescription medications.

✓ *For a second opinion, understand why you are going and be prepared.* Call ahead and find out what information the consulting physician needs prior to your visit. Make sure it gets there, and bring a copy with you on that visit, just in case.

✓ *Informed consent is the idea that patients have a right to be provided with information* and a level of understanding to weigh the benefits, risks, and alternatives of having any treatment or procedure done. Then the patient can make an informed decision regarding his or her care.

✓ *You don't always need to see your doctor for simple problems.* Go to www.familydoctor.org to help you decide when to seek care. Even if you feel perfectly well, definitely get preventive tests done to stay healthy.

PART THREE:

Do the Right Thing Regularly and Repeatedly

> A little neglect may breed mischief: for want of a nail the shoe was lost; for want of a shoe the horse was lost; and for want of a horse the rider was lost.
>
> — Benjamin Franklin[46]

THE PRUDENT APPROACH TO STAYING HEALTHY

Should we actively search for good health? Should we be proactive in looking for signs and symptoms of illness even though we feel completely fine? Our bodies are amazingly complex and dynamic machines. We are able to tolerate different environments and climates, nourish ourselves with a variety of foods, and perform a large number of physical tasks, all as the body keeps itself running on a daily basis. Cells grow, regenerate, and die in a controlled fashion. Organs replenish themselves and compensate, despite what we expose them to. It's a true wonder that our bodies don't break down more often.

Perhaps that's why many of us get an annual "general check-up" or physical examination to make sure everything is okay. If you like to have a physical examination, you are not alone. A 2002 article in the Annals of Internal Medicine found that a majority of the public still feels that a comprehensive physical examination is necessary even though recent

> *A majority of the public still feels that a comprehensive physical examination is necessary even though recent medical evidence and guidelines do not recommend it.*

medical evidence and guidelines do not recommend it.[47] It may not be too surprising to you that when you have a physical, nothing significant is usually discovered.

The study also found that patients were less willing to have a physical or a recommended screening test when costs were mentioned. With increasing health care costs, you can expect to pay more. The question is, then, should you have a physical? If so, when should you get one and what should you ask for?

Manage your body like you manage your car. You're told to take your car in for important scheduled services every few thousand miles. But if your car is running well, aside from these critical minor and major services you wouldn't dream of dropping by the mechanic's garage just to make sure everything was okay, would you?

Assuming you feel well, have no areas or symptoms of concern, and don't fit any of the following recommendations, a general check-up for the sake of it might not be very valuable. If, however, you would just feel better by getting one, by all means get one. Just realize that there is no scientific evidence beyond the recommendations we review which shows that routine physicals help save lives.

If our bodies came with a maintenance manual, it would list the following guidelines as absolutely critical. The prudent approach to staying healthy means regularly and systematically looking for potential health problems and catching them early enough so they don't impact your life. You will need to undergo screening tests that vary depending on your age and gender. The older you are, the more likely it is that you will need mammograms, colonoscopies, and prostate examinations, for example.

The younger you are, the less likely it is that you need to see a doctor or have any tests. Of course, there are exceptions, i.e., routine Pap smears/pelvic exams that screen for cervical cancer and sexually transmitted diseases.

Remember: Life happens. Disease happens. Feeling healthy is not a good reason to skip these vital and indicated screening tests.

If you do get the recommended testing done, don't be surprised if you aren't offered a chest x-ray and urine test. Although they were routine in the past, medical research showed that these tests did not save lives and instead caused unnecessary additional procedures, especially in patients who had no complaints or symptoms. Therefore, these tests won't be ordered unless you or your doctor has some concerns.

Remember: Life happens. Disease happens. Feeling healthy is not a good reason to skip these vital and indicated screening tests. Admittedly there is nothing glamorous, exciting, sexy, or even fun about doing these boring and mundane interventions consistently and regularly — but much like putting on your seatbelt, they have been proven time and time again to save lives. Each of us has only one life to live. Make sure you actively search for good health to make the most of it.

Real Life Example

> Mr. Smith went to his doctor. He was a sixty-five-year-old man who took no medications and had no medical problems. His last office visit was five years ago for a physical. He didn't feel compelled to come in sooner because he felt fine. He didn't smoke or drink. He exercised regularly. His weight and blood pressure were in the normal range. Unfortunately the rectal exam revealed a rock-hard

prostate, classic for advanced prostate cancer. Blood work strongly suggested that his prostate cancer had spread beyond the prostate gland.

Perhaps had he been examined and screened regularly, even though he was healthy, the cancer might have been discovered at an earlier stage. Early detection might have simply involved prostate surgery or local radiation treatment to eradicate the cancerous growth, and then periodic follow up. Instead, because he has metastatic disease, Mr. Smith now sees a urologist for a prostate biopsy, sees an oncologist for chemotherapy regularly, and a radiation oncologist for radiation therapy. The treatments cause him to have hot flashes. His out-of-pocket costs have increased dramatically as he pays for additional office visits, treatments, medications, and procedures. His quality of life suffers as he undergoes powerful therapies which, in the end, might not be enough to improve his long-term prognosis and survival.

To stay healthy, wise patients know to ask for recommended screening tests even if they are doing the right things and have no symptoms, problems, or concerns. The American Cancer Society's *Cancer Prevention and Early Detection Facts & Figures 2005* noted that at least half of all cancer deaths could be prevented if patients adopted a healthier lifestyle and got the necessary screening tests.

To stay healthy, follow the latest guidelines from the American Diabetes Association, American Heart Association, and the American Cancer Society. Necessary tests and interventions include cholesterol tests, pap smears, breast exams, mammograms, prostate exams, and screening for high blood pressure and colon cancer. Since insurance plans generally try to promote preventive health, these tests are often covered. Use these benefits.

At least half of all cancer deaths could be prevented if patients adopted a healthier lifestyle and got the necessary screening tests.

Furthermore, make an effort to understand the recommendations from the U.S. Preventive Services Task Force (USPSTF). This independent committee of primary care and preventive physicians periodically reviews the latest medical research and recommends tests and screening methods that have scientifically been shown to make a difference. As a result, its recommendations are the most conservative of any national organization.

Since these are all national guidelines, patients should not have a problem getting their insurance plans to cover these services. To help you figure out which tests to ask for, I've included a summary of the suggested screening tests divided by age group and gender at the end of this section.

With this information, you will now have to make a choice. You can wait for disease and illness to develop and then deal with the consequences. (In the case of cancer, this could mean surgery, chemotherapy, radiation, or other treatments to improve your odds of survival.) Or, you could go on the offensive, search actively for disease, and find it early. Caught at an early stage, the treatments might be fewer and less intense. Your chance for survival will be much higher, and your quality of life maintained. It is entirely up to you.

AMERICAN CANCER SOCIETY (ACS)

In 2004, cancer was the leading cause of death in the United States, surpassing heart disease for the first time. Despite the many advances in chemotherapy and radiation treatments, chances of long-term survival are still better the earlier the cancer is detected. By the time patients begin developing symptoms like weight loss or fatigue, or discover a lump, the cancer may have already spread.

Although one can decrease the risk of cancer by not smoking, maintaining a healthy weight, exercising, and eating well, cancer can still occur. Even children and young adults who often haven't had enough time to adopt unhealthy lifestyles can develop cancer. There are no excuses. Get checked. Additional up-to-date information can be found at www.cancer.org.

CANCER GUIDELINES FOR WOMEN

Cervical Cancer Screening

For women, the American Cancer Society recommends the Pap smear to screen for cervical cancer. Women should begin having the test regularly when they first become sexually active or at age twenty-one, whichever comes first.[48] Women should get the Pap test every year, or the new liquid Pap test every other year. If a woman has three normal Pap smears in a row, she can then have a Pap test or the liquid test every two to three years.[49]

The Pap smear consists of a pelvic examination where the doctor first examines the vagina, then places either a plastic or metal speculum into the vagina to allow him to see the cervix. Many women find the insertion of the speculum in the vagina uncomfortable. The doctor then takes a couple of swabs and/or a small wooden spatula (as long, but not as wide as a tongue depressor) to rub off some cervical cells to send to a pathologist for analysis.

The speculum is removed. The doctor will then insert his gloved fingers into the vagina to manually feel the uterus and ovaries. Doctors will often do a rectal exam as well, to ensure that there are no abnormal rectal growths.

To get the best results, the Pap smear is best performed when a woman is not having her period, has not had sex the night before, and does not have a yeast or other infection. Any of these situations can make the samples difficult to interpret and may require a repeat Pap smear.

The risk of developing cervical cancer is thought to be higher if the human papilloma virus (HPV) is present in the cervix. HPV is sexually transmitted and patients often have no symptoms. Women who have had three normal Pap smears in a row can get tested every three years with an HPV test and Pap smear or can opt to be tested every two to three years with a Pap or newer liquid Pap (ACS).[50] Women thirty or older should ask their doctor whether they perform HPV testing with their Pap smear, since HPV testing is relatively new. At this time it is only recommended for women aged thirty and older.

Multiple studies have shown that there is a big misconception about Pap smears and pelvic examinations. They are not the same.

In the future, HPV infection may be less likely. Vaccines that would protect against the four types of HPV which are responsible for 70 percent of cervical cancers are currently under development.[51] In 2006, the FDA approved the first vaccine that decreases the risk of getting an HPV infection (see the section on immunizations).

Multiple studies have shown that there is a big misconception about Pap smears and pelvic examinations. They are not the same. Doctors use a plastic or metal speculum for either test. But if a physician does not use a swab or wooden spatula to rub off cervical cells, a Pap smear was not done. In one study of two hundred women who had pelvic examinations done in the emergency room, nearly 60 percent believed that a Pap smear had been done while only 10 percent correctly noted that a Pap had not been done.[52] The remaining 30 percent either weren't sure or skipped the question.

When a Pap smear is done, doctors may or may not also be checking for sexually transmitted diseases (STDs) like gonorrhea or chlamydia. If you are concerned about your risk, then tell your doctor to check for these bacteria in addition to the Pap smear (see USPSTF section).

Unfortunately, there are no recommended tests to screen for ovarian cancer, but research continues to try and find reliable tests. A doctor's examination of the ovaries as part of the pelvic exam can help detect abnormalities.

Breast Cancer Screening

The lifetime risk of a woman developing breast cancer is one in seven. *One common misconception is that breast cancer occurs primarily in women with a family history. In fact, the vast majority of breast cancers occur in women with no family history. The other misconception is that many women feel as they get older that their risk of developing breast cancer decreases. Their risk of breast cancer actually increases.*

The vast majority of breast cancers occur in women with no family history.

With increased awareness, thanks in part to the pink ribbons, the annual Susan G. Komen Race for the Cure, the breast cancer research stamp, and breast cancer awareness month, you would expect that women would be well informed about breast cancer. You'd think women would get regular mammograms, perform breast self-exams, and have regular clinical exams performed by physicians. An October 2005 article in the *New England Journal of Medicine* found that in fact mammography was largely responsible for the improvement in breast cancer survival over the past twenty-five years.

Despite this, women are not getting mammograms as suggested. In 2002, only 62 percent of women forty and older reported having a mammogram within the previous year. The number decreased to less than 40 percent in women without insurance.[53] Another study showed that only two-thirds of women forty and older in New Hampshire received mammograms annually or biannually even though 97 percent had health insurance and over half (61 percent) were college educated.[54]

Screening for breast cancer begins by doing a self breast examination monthly. Learn how to perform a breast self exam (BSE) correctly at www.komen.org/bse. To be completely thorough, also get a mammogram if it is indicated for your age group. Often, mammograms detect breast cancer at a much earlier stage and well before a lump is large enough to be felt by yourself or a doctor. Mammograms can also detect growths too deep in the breast to be felt by anyone. However, performing a breast self-exam regularly is equally as important, since some breast cancers cannot be identified by mammography.

Women are recommended to get mammograms annually starting at age forty.[55] Make sure that your mammogram is performed by an accredited facility and the results are interpreted by qualified radiologists. Refer to the FDA Center for Devices and Radiological Health at www.fda.gov/cdrh and look for the mammogram program.[56]

If you feel a lump, or your breast just doesn't feel right to you, see your doctor right away even if you had a normal mammogram recently. Sometimes growths can occur and you may need another mammogram or other additional tests like an ultrasound.

Newer digital mammograms are on the horizon. Preliminary results have shown that these mammograms may be more effective in detecting tumors in women with dense breasts, who are not menopausal, or are under fifty years of age. And for women who do not fit into these categories, digital mammography was found to be equally as effective as traditional film-based mammograms.[57]

In 2007, the American Cancer Society recommended breast MRIs as another way of screening for breast cancer in women who were considered high risk for developing the disease. (A lifetime risk of 20 percent or higher is considered high risk.) Your doctor has a variety of tools that can predict this risk. One is available from the National Cancer Institute at www.cancer.gov/bcrisktool.

If you are considered high risk, ask your doctor whether a breast MRI is right for you and whether your hospital can perform the test. It may be a while before your local MRI facility will have the appropriate setup and radiologists trained to interpret the breast MRI correctly. The breast MRI is to be used with a mammogram and should not replace mammograms. Women at high risk for breast cancer should consider getting both a mammogram and a breast MRI at age thirty. Women with a risk of 15 to 20 percent should ask their doctor whether a breast MRI is a good idea.

Regardless of whether you use traditional film-based or digital mammograms, if a mammogram is indicated for your age group get it done.

Ovarian Cancer Screening

One of the most feared cancers for many women is ovarian cancer, which occurs in one out of sixty-eight women.[58] Unfortunately, research has not shown that ultrasound screenings for the disease are particularly helpful. The blood test CA 125, which is used to check for recurrence in ovarian cancer patients, unfortunately isn't a good test either for screening the general public. Nevertheless, research continues, and perhaps one day there will be a good test to detect an illness that is diagnosed late and can be present with vague symptoms like abdominal bloating and fullness.

CANCER GUIDELINES FOR MEN

Testicular Cancer Screening

Testicular cancer is the most common cancer among young men. Unlike many of the tests discussed here, you do not need a doctor or special test to screen for it. Check yourself monthly in the shower and see if you feel any abnormal lumps or bumps in the testicle. The testicle is usually smooth. A good article with diagrams and explanations is at the FDA Consumer Magazine page, www.fda.gov/fdac. Search for testicular self exam (TSE). Men should begin self-screening at age twenty.[59]

Prostate Cancer Screening

The American Cancer Society recommends that men with a family history of prostate cancer (i.e. in a close relative) or who are African American get a prostate examination, a rectal exam, and a prostate-specific antigen (PSA) blood test every year starting at age forty-five and possibly even at forty if multiple family members have had the disease.[60] Otherwise, all men should be offered these tests starting at age fifty. Individuals in this latter group should also know that they may or may not benefit from testing.

The reason for this uncertainty is controversy surrounding the PSA blood test. Originally, the PSA test was used in prostate cancer patients as a way of seeing if the cancer had returned or was advancing. Typically, after treatment, the PSA would be less than 0.1. If the cancer returned, the PSA would start to rise. The PSA level, however, can be measured in all men. The normal range is 0 to 4 ng/ml, and an elevated value could be the result of an enlarged but normal prostate or a small prostate cancer which will never be life threatening.[61] Used in the past exclusively on prostate cancer patients, the PSA is now being used as a screening test.

As a result, many men may undergo biopsies or treatments like surgery or radiation for cancers that in fact may not shorten their lives. Although the National Cancer Institute is currently evaluating the importance of PSA screening and digital rectal examination in saving lives in its Prostate, Lung, Colorectal, and Ovarian Cancer Screening Trial

(PLCO trial), results will not be available for several years. Even the doctor who discovered the PSA test has expressed his concern that the extensive use of PSA testing is not warranted.[62]

No major scientific or medical organizations, including the American Cancer Society, National Comprehensive Cancer Network, American Urological Association, U.S. Preventive Services Task Force, American College of Physicians-American Society of Internal Medicine, National Cancer Institute, American Academy of Family Physicians, or American College of Preventive Medicine currently advocate routine testing for prostate cancer at this time.[63]

The conclusion? Have a frank discussion with your doctor about the pros and cons of screening for prostate cancer. Since current research is not conclusive, you and your doctor can decide which is more harmful: having potentially unnecessary tests, procedures, or treatments or missing something completely by not looking for a problem. The choice is ultimately yours.

CANCER GUIDELINES FOR WOMEN AND MEN

Colon Cancer Screening

Despite being the third leading cause of cancer deaths, the majority of patients do not get screened for colon cancer.

Despite being the third leading cause of cancer deaths, the majority of patients do not get screened for colon cancer. This is probably because the screening tests, which include flexible sigmoidoscopy, colonoscopy, barium enema, and stool testing, are quite unappealing. One study found that only 14 percent of eligible patients had the combination of stool testing and sigmoidoscopy, while only 3 percent had a colonoscopy.[64] Although they're less invasive, virtual colonoscopies are not recommended.

The American Cancer Society estimates that 90 percent of colon cancer cases and deaths could be prevented if everyone over fifty practiced a healthy lifestyle and received regular screening, including annual stool testing with a flexible sigmoidoscopy every five years, a colonoscopy every ten years, or a barium enema every five years.[65] The risk of doing nothing is real, since for both men and women the lifetime risk of developing either colon or rectal cancer is about one in eighteen.[66]

For both men and women the lifetime risk of developing either colon or rectal cancer is about one in eighteen.

Sigmoidoscopy and colonoscopy procedures are similar except that the former examines the lower third of the colon (the sigmoid) and the latter the entire colon. The colonoscopy, however, requires that a patient drink much more laxative and be put under sedation. Both the sigmoidoscope and colonoscope are slightly wider than a dime and two to three feet in length. A small port in the scope allows a physician to biopsy any suspicious growths seen in the colon. Fiber optics in the scopes allow the doctor to see the colon through a viewfinder or on a video monitor. The procedure typically takes thirty to sixty minutes, depending on the individual case.

A barium enema also requires that a patient drink a laxative to clean out the colon. Unlike the other procedures, a white dye, called barium, is inserted into the rectum and coats the colon. X-rays are taken and radiologists can determine if any growths are present. If abnormalities are seen, patients may need to undergo a sigmoidoscopy, colonoscopy, or biopsy.

Patients without a family history should start with these procedures at age fifty. Those with a first-degree relative (parent, sibling, or child), two family members, or a relative diagnosed before age fifty with colon cancer are at higher risk and should discuss with their doctor the indications for screening before age fifty.[67]

Lung Cancer

Unfortunately, there are no screening tests for lung cancer, which one in thirteen men, and one in eighteen women, will be diagnosed with.[68] It was once thought that annual chest x-rays would detect lung cancer sooner in asymptomatic patients, but research has shown that not to be the case. Although there is always ongoing research to find new tests and techniques, there is no definitive test for lung cancer at this time.

AMERICAN HEART ASSOCIATION (AHA)

Heart Disease

The American Heart Association's recommendations aim to help individuals decrease their risk of developing heart disease and stroke, which, until cancer recently surpassed them, were the leading causes of death and disability in America. Even if a person doesn't die suddenly from a massive heart attack or devastating stroke, his or her quality of life can decrease greatly. A heart attack can damage the heart muscle, causing congestive heart failure. With a weakened heart that's unable to circulate blood effectively, individuals complain of fatigue with exertion, shortness of breath with simple physical tasks, or leg swelling. Patients who suffer from strokes might have mild symptoms like some weakness in an arm or leg. Unfortunately, strokes can also be devastating, damaging the speech center and silencing a person permanently or damaging the swallow center, forever causing the patient to rely on a feeding tube. We don't get to choose how mild or severe our heart attacks or strokes might be. To minimize your risk, make sure your blood pressure and cholesterol are in the desirable range and that you do not smoke. Learn more at www.americanheart.org.

High Blood Pressure

The American Heart Association and the Joint National Commission on Hypertension recommend that everyone should ideally have a blood pressure less than 120/80. Check your blood pressure periodically even if you feel well, as high blood pressure, also known as hypertension, is quite common. Use the automatic blood pressure machines available at drug stores or attend a health fair and have it evaluated. Check your blood pressure more often if it is greater than 120/80. Blood pressures between 120–140/80–90 are considered in the pre-high blood pressure range. Consider consulting your doctor when it is in the pre-high blood pressure range. Definitely see your doctor if your blood pressure is consistently greater than 140/90 to discuss treatment options and interventions. Either number is important; if your top number (systolic) is always over 140 or the bottom number (diastolic) is routinely over 90, see your doctor.

One out of three of adults have high blood pressure, and a third of those people are unaware that they have it.[69] Known as the silent killer, high blood pressure does not cause symptoms as it quietly damages the body. Left untreated, high blood pressure can lead to heart attack, congestive heart failure, stroke, and kidney failure.

One of the misconceptions many patients have is that you need to be overweight or obese to have high blood pressure. Another is that you need to be older. Hypertension can occur at any age and patients with a family history should be monitoring their blood pressure periodically. And don't fool yourself into thinking that your blood pressure is only high when you see the doctor. Known as "white coat

One out of three of adults have high blood pressure, and a third of those people are unaware that they have it.

hypertension," this phenomenon refers to patients whose blood pressure is higher in the physician's office than when it is measured at home. While many patients claim to have this condition, very few go and check themselves regularly away from the doctor's office to convince themselves that their blood pressure is in the safe range. In fact, the only time they record their blood pressure readings is when they see the doctor. Could it be that they actually have high blood pressure?

If you and your doctor decide it's prudent to take medication for high blood pressure, you should still check your blood pressure regularly. The goal is the same: ideally, you want a blood pressure reading of less than 120/80 but at least less than 140/90. For patients with diabetes, kidney disease, or heart disease the target should be less than 130/85.

Remember, *merely taking blood pressure medication doesn't mean your high blood pressure is well controlled. You still need to monitor it regularly.* You might surprise yourself. With hard work, dietary changes, exercise, and medication your blood pressure may consistently be less than 120/80. At that point, ask your doctor if reducing some of your medication might be appropriate. Never adjust or quit taking medication without checking with your doctor. If you are having side effects, let him know; there are many alternative drugs. It is far better to monitor your progress, adjust your medications, and continue feeling great than regret what steps you *should have* taken after suffering a heart attack or stroke.

High Cholesterol

We have all heard that having high blood cholesterol is not good. But it's not just cholesterol that's important. Other factors play a role in predicting your chance of developing heart disease or stroke. Find out your likelihood of developing or dying of a heart attack over a ten-year period using the cholesterol risk calculator at the National Heart Lung Institute website: www.nhlbi.nih.gov/guidelines/cholesterol. This calculator uses six factors to determine your risk: age, gender, smoking status, blood pressure, total cholesterol, and good cholesterol. The results are only meant for patients over twenty years of age who have never been diagnosed with heart disease or diabetes. You will need to have a recent blood pressure reading as well as your total cholesterol and HDL (good) cholesterol to use the calculator.

The calculation is based on the information and findings from the famous Framingham Heart Study. This research study initially started in 1948 and followed a group of over five thousand adults, ages thirty to sixty-two, with extensive physical examinations, history taking, and blood work every two years to determine risk factors and patterns for heart disease.[70] In 1971, the study followed a similar number of the original participants' adult children and their spouses.

Though the data was based on thousands of people over a period of years, the calculation may not be entirely accurate for individuals who are non-white (the study was performed on people living in Framingham, Massachusetts, which at the time of the study was predominately Caucasian). Nevertheless, we can thank the study for our current understanding that addressing high blood pressure, high cholesterol, smoking, obesity, diabetes, and physical inactivity decreases the risk for heart disease.

In order to know if you're at risk, get your cholesterol checked, including your total cholesterol, triglycerides, HDL (good) cholesterol, and LDL (bad) cholesterol. And remember that while an individual cannot change risk factors like age or gender, other risk factors for heart disease are modifiable. Blood pressure and cholesterol can be lowered. For one thing, people can decide whether or not to smoke, and whether or not to eat well. If, after taking the test, you discover that your risk is 10 to 20 percent or 20 percent or higher, you should check with your doctor. He may suggest that diet and exercise are enough or if a cholesterol-lowering medication needs to be prescribed to further decrease your risk.

AMERICAN DIABETES ASSOCIATION (ADA)

Diabetes

According to the American Diabetes Association, an epidemic of diabetes is occurring not only in adults, but also in children and teenagers. *In the United States, diabetes is the leading cause of blindness and kidney failure requiring dialysis.* Diabetics are also at increased risk for heart attacks and limb amputations. The good news is that individuals with a family history of diabetes may not be destined to develop diabetes. Research has shown that patients with a family history can decrease their risk with a program of diet and exercise.

A person with a fasting blood sugar of 126 mg/dl, tested on two different occasions, is considered as having diabetes.

Aside from patients with a family history, who else should be screened for diabetes? The ADA recommends that people forty-five years old and older, and particularly those with a body mass index (BMI) of 25 kg/m² or greater, which is considered overweight, should receive a fasting blood sugar test.[71] A person with a fasting blood sugar of 126 mg/dl, tested on two different occasions, is considered as having diabetes.

In people over forty-five with fasting blood sugar levels of less than 126 mg/dl, the test should be repeated every three years. Testing should also be considered for individuals younger than forty-five who may have the following characteristics: [72]

➤ Have high blood pressure

➤ Are overweight or obese

➤ Are a member of a high-risk group (i.e. African Americans, Latinos, Asian Americans, Native Americans, or Pacific Islanders)

➤ Are women with histories of diabetes during pregnancy or

following delivery of a baby greater than nine pounds

➤ Have a first-degree relative with diabetes (i.e. parent or sibling)

If you fit any of the above criteria, even if you feel well, be sure to get your blood sugar (glucose) checked periodically. Read more about pre-diabetes, diabetes, and how to prevent these conditions at www.diabetes.org.

By the way: to calculate your body mass index, or BMI, go to www.cdc.gov and search for BMI. You will need to know your height and weight. If you wish to calculate it by hand, the formula is:

weight (in pounds)/height ^{2} (in inches) x 703

or

weight (in kilograms)/height ^{2} (in meters)

Obesity is defined as a body mass index of 30 or greater, while overweight is defined as a BMI of 25 to 29.9. BMI is meant to be a quick and easy tool for you and your doctor to determine how your weight compares with that of the general public. About 30 percent of adults twenty years and older are considered obese.[73] These adults are at greater risk for diabetes.

About 30 percent of adults twenty years and older are considered obese.

U.S. PREVENTIVE SERVICES TASK FORCE (USPSTF)

Medical research continues at an astonishing rate. Existing tests continue to be refined, screening guidelines are constantly revised, and new technologies are introduced. Determining whether these interventions and new technologies work and save lives is the role of the U.S. Preventive Services Task Force.

Consisting of a panel of independent experts in primary care and preventive medicine, the USPSTF's recommendations are considered the "gold standard" for determining which clinical services are preventive.[74] They review and look at various screening tests and preventive medications to determine whether there's proof these interventions work and that the benefits they provide outweigh the potential harm.

USPSTF indicates how strongly it recommends a particular method with a letter grade designation (A, B, C, D, and I). An A recommendation means that USPSTF strongly recommends that doctors provide a particular service to eligible patients. A B rating is simply a recommendation. A C means the task force makes no recommendation, since it has found the difference between the risk and benefit provided by a particular method too close for recommendation. A D rating means the group recommends against providing for a particular intervention. An I recommendation indicates that there is not enough evidence to determine whether to recommend for or against a particular procedure.[75]

The USPSTF recommendations tend to be the most conservative of any national organization, because they look for interventions that have proven benefits backed by research. Therefore, promising new technologies and tests that are yet unproven (and at times remain unproven or shown to be no better than existing tests) will not be recommended. As a result, the USPSTF's guidelines may lag behind those of other organizations. But because they set such a high standard before recommending a particular treatment, insurers should cover the tests and procedures rated A and B.

Below, I highlight only the USPSTF's strongly recommended and recommended services (the As and Bs) from the *2005 Guide to Clinical Preventive Services*. Look to see which ones apply to you. Additional information and recommendations can be found at the Agency for

Healthcare Research and Quality at www.ahrq.gov. Find the U.S. Preventive Services Task Force link.

Grade A Recommendations

Both Men and Women

➤ Screen all adults for tobacco use and provide treatment for those who use these products.

➤ Encourage the use of aspirin in appropriate patients to decrease their risk of heart disease. (Your doctor can advise you of the appropriate dosage).

➤ Screen patients older than eighteen for high blood pressure.

➤ Screen men over thirty-five and women over forty-five for high cholesterol and treat when appropriate.

➤ Screen patients fifty and older for colon cancer.

➤ Screen for syphilis in patients at increased risk.

Women

➤ Screen all women who are three- to four-months pregnant with a urine culture for bacteria.

➤ Screen women who are sexually active and have a cervix (i.e. it has not been removed) for cervical cancer.

➤ Routinely screen sexually active women twenty-five years of age and younger for Chlamydia.

➤ Screen pregnant women at their first visit for hepatitis B, Rh incompatibility testing, and syphilis.

Grade B Recommendations

Men and Women

> ➤ Screen for diabetes in patients with high blood pressure or high cholesterol.

> ➤ Clinical practices with programs that can accurately diagnose, treat, and follow-up should screen for depression.

> ➤ Offer dietary and behavioral counseling to those with high cholesterol or other risk factors for heart disease or diabetes.

> ➤ Screen for obesity and offer counseling or behavioral therapies to promote weight loss.

> ➤ Screen and counsel to decrease misuse of alcohol.

Men

> ➤ One-time screen with ultrasound for abdominal aortic aneurysm in a sixty-five to seventy-five-year-old man who smoked 100 or more cigarettes.

Women

> ➤ Promote breast feeding.

> ➤ Provide mammograms with or without breast examination for women age forty and older every one to two years.

> ➤ Promote breast cancer prevention in women at high risk by prescribing preventive medication.

> ➤ Routinely screen women sixty-five years and older for osteoporosis. Screen high risk women at age sixty.

Children

> ➤ Ensure that preschool children older than six months receive oral fluoride if their water supply is deficient in fluoride in order to prevent cavities.

➤ Screen children younger than age five for amblyopia (lazy eye), strabismus (cross eyes), and problems with visual acuity.

IMMUNIZATIONS AND VACCINATIONS

Measles. Mumps. German measles. Polio. Most of us have not had personal experience with these illnesses since the implementation of the respective vaccines. Before the measles vaccine, annually there were about 450,000 cases of measles, which resulted in 450 deaths.[76] Since the licensing of the vaccine in 1963, the number of cases has dropped by 98 percent, with only small outbreaks occurring in communities that declined the vaccine; among high school and college students who were inadequately immunized; or among travelers visiting countries where the illness is still common.[77]

One of the first vaccinations was performed in 1796 by Dr. Edward Jenner. He was trying to protect patients from smallpox, which for many was lethal and for others left disfiguring scars.[78] He observed that many of the women who milked cows developed an illness called cowpox, but never developed the more deadly smallpox. He theorized that exposure to cowpox protected the individual. So Dr. Jenner inoculated a young boy, illustrating that he was protected from getting the deadly smallpox.

Aside from preventing illness in an individual, immunizations, done on a massive scale, can decrease the number of cases within the community. About 150 years after Dr. Jenner's experiment, the World Health Assembly adopted a goal to eradicate smallpox with a worldwide vaccination program. By 1977, the last case of smallpox was noted. By 1980, the World Health Organization reported that smallpox was gone, and thus, routine vaccination was no longer necessary. This is one example of how a successful vaccination program can reduce or even eliminate an otherwise harmful or fatal disease.

Vaccines come in two forms. They either contain a component of the virus or bacterium that is inactive; or one that is attenuated or weakened. In an inactive vaccine, either the organism was killed or portions of the organism were used. In the case of attenuated, or "live," vaccines, the organism is still active, but does not result in severe infection.

In either case, the vaccine works much like a fire drill: it stimulates the immune system so that if the individual is exposed to the real infection, the immune system will respond more quickly and more vigorously to eradicate the organism before it becomes a potentially serious problem.

Although most vaccines are covered by insurance, periodic changes in vaccine recommendations, as well as the development of new vaccine combinations (to minimize the number of injections given) may result in times when they are not covered. This happens when your doctor does not get reimbursed for purchasing the vaccine and administering it to you and thus loses money on each vaccine given. You may end up paying for a vaccine out of pocket in that scenario. The pneumococcal vaccine, which requires a total of four shots at $58.75 each, would total $235.[79]

However, there are sometimes ways to mitigate these costs. For example, children who are eligible for Medicaid, have no health insurance, or have health insurance which does not cover vaccines, are covered by the federal government's Vaccines for Children program, which provides recommended immunizations to children up to and through age eighteen at little to no out-of pocket cost. Learn more at www.cdc.gov/vaccines/programs/vfc.

Vaccines decrease the chance of missing work or becoming ill, lower the need for medications or hospitalization for influenza or pneumonia, and may prevent contracting an antibiotic-resistant bacteria.

New vaccines continue to be developed. These days, children born in America can also add varicella, or chickenpox, to the list of illnesses they will never have to endure. Future generations of women will decrease their risk of developing cervical cancer and genital warts with a vaccine to protect against a variety of human papilloma viruses. Many older adults will be spared from an extremely painful, and at times disabling, skin condition, shingles, by getting immunized.

Fortunately, there aren't many vaccines that adults need. To ensure that you are up to date, learn more about the vaccines and the diseases they are protecting you against at the National Immunization Program (NIP) website at www. cdc.gov/vaccines. Access the recommend adult immunization schedule as well as one for children and adolescents. These are updated annually. Vaccines still have a role in the twenty-first century and wise patients should consider getting them.

Vaccines still have a role in the twenty-first century and wise patients should consider getting them.

Immunization Guidelines

Tetanus

For adults, the tetanus vaccine is given once every ten years as a booster. It protects an individual from Clostridium tetani, which is found in soil and in the fecal material of animal feces. Once clostridium tetani enters a person's body, typically through a wound, it can cause lockjaw, difficulty swallowing, muscle spasms, and even death (in over 10 percent of cases).[80]

Hepatitis B

This vaccine consists of an inactive viral component and requires a series of three shots over a period of six months. Currently any baby born in the United States is started on Hepatitis B immunizations. It protects individuals from developing hepatitis or inflammation of the liver. Chronic irritation or hepatitis can progress to cirrhosis, liver failure, or liver cancer. Hepatitis B can be transmitted by sexual activity or intrave-nous drug use.

Pertussis (Whooping Cough)

Already given routinely to infants, a new vaccine has been approved for older children and adults to protect them from the *Bortella pertussis* bacteria, which causes whooping cough. Should babies acquire it, it can be lethal as the persistent cough tires the baby, causes difficulty breath-ing, and can make them turn blue. Although older children and adults can handle the cough, the infection can cause them to cough for weeks or months.

Meningiococcus

Meningiococcus is one of three bacteria that can cause meningitis (the other two are H. influenzae and pneumococcus, both of which can also be guarded against by vaccines). Although meningitis is rare and more common among infants, about half the cases are in children fif-teen and older. Meningitis kills over 20 percent of patients aged fifteen to twenty-four who contract the illness.[81]

Currently, eleven to twelve year olds, those entering high school, and freshmen entering college are recommended to have the vaccine. It cost $82 in 2005.[82]

Human Papilloma Virus

Human Papilloma Virus, or HPV, is a very common sexually trans-mitted disease that can cause cervical cancer in women. In 2006 the FDA approved a vaccine that can protect women from four of the forty types of HPV. Of these four, two types cause 70 percent of cervical can-cer and the other two cause 90 percent of genital warts.[83] The vaccine is a series of three shots given over a six-month period and is recom-mended routinely for females between eleven and twenty-six.

Unlike other vaccines which protect individuals from infection, this vaccine decreases a person's risk of developing cancer. In the United States, nearly 10,000 women are diagnosed with cervical cancer every year and 3,700 will die from the disease.

Pneumococcus

Prior to the development of a vaccine that protected against Streptococcus pneumoniae, the bacteria annually caused over 700 cases of meningitis, 13,000 cases of blood infections, over 5,000,000 ear infections, and 200 deaths in children under five from invasive disease.[84] Among adults in 2000, there were about 135,000 hospitalizations due to pneumonia, and 60,000 cases of invasive disease, which included 3,300 cases of meningitis. Of those patients with the aggressive invasive disease, 14 percent were fatal.[85]

The type of vaccine administered varies depending on the age of the patient. For children, the vaccine is a series of shots given between the age of two to twenty-three months and is known as the pneumococcal conjugate vaccine (PCV). Other children may also get this vaccine at a later age if they have certain medical conditions. The pneumococcal polysaccharide vaccine (PPV) is recommended for adults sixty-five and older or who have other medical conditions. PPV is also given to children over the age of two with chronic illnesses.

Over time, this bacterium has become resistant to more antibiotics. This alone may be a good enough reason to get vaccinated. It is better not to get the illness rather than hope the right antibiotic is used should you get ill. To find out if you should get this vaccine, check with your doctor.

Influenza

Given annually in the fall, this vaccine is made from a killed virus. Since the flu virus changes year to year, a new formulation for the vaccine is developed annually to reflect these changes. It is estimated that anywhere from 5 to 20 percent of the population contracts the flu every year. Over 200,000 people are hospitalized, and 36,000 die.[86]

Like the pneumococcal vaccine, the flu shot is recommended for patients with respiratory problems like asthma or emphysema. It is also recommend for women who will be in their second or third trimester of pregnancy during the flu season, children between six months and fifty-nine months, caregivers of those children, and adults fifty years of age and older.[87]

HAPPY BIRTHDAY TO YOU

Life is truly unpredictable. I have had friends pass away suddenly at young ages (under thirty) due to cancer, sudden unexplained deaths, and accidents. These were all healthy individuals; no one expected their lives to be cut short so soon.

Life is precious and too often we assume and take for granted our good health. Anything can happen to us at any time.

As a physician, I periodically see patients with serious medical problems at a young age. As a result, despite most of us groaning about becoming a year older, I see it as a true blessing. Life is precious and too often we assume and take for granted our good health. Anything can happen to us at any time.

To ensure that you stay healthy, I've summarized below some age-specific guidelines. It would be nice if each of us had an owner's manual that told us which tests should be done, and when, for us to stay healthy. It would be better if our bodies, like our cars, had a little maintenance light that flashed on the dashboard when we were due for vital screening interventions. The closest and easiest reminder we have is our birthdays. Every year, review the age-specific guidelines. See which ones apply to you, consult with your doctor, and give yourself a gift every year. Make sure you are actively looking to stay healthy by getting the right tests done. Happy Birthday to you!

Age-Specific Guidelines

Twenty to thirty-nine years old

- ➤ Patients older than eighteen should be screened for high blood pressure (USPSTF).

- ➤ Men over thirty-five and women over forty-five should have their cholesterol checked and treated when appropriate (USPSTF).

- ➤ Patients at risk for heart disease should take aspirin to decrease their risk of heart disease (USPSTF).

- ➤ When they first become sexually active, or at age twenty-one, whichever is earlier, women should have a Pap smear every year (or the newer liquid Pap test every other year). If a woman has three normal Pap smears in a row, she can then have a Pap test or liquid Pap test every two to three years. Women age thirty and older can ask for HPV testing during the Pap smear. Women in this age group who have had three normal Pap smears in a row should be tested every three years with an HPV test with Pap, or can opt for testing every two to three with a Pap or newer liquid Pap (ACS).

- ➤ Sexually active women ages twenty-five and younger should be routinely screened for Chlamydia (USPSTF).

- ➤ Patients with high blood pressure or high cholesterol should be checked for diabetes (USPSTF). Individuals who are members of a high risk ethnic group (African Americans, Latinos, Asian Americans, Pacific Islanders, or Native Americans), individuals who have a body mass index of twenty-five or greater (overweight), individuals with first-degree relatives with diabetes, or women who during pregnancy developed gestational diabetes or delivered a nine-pound baby should also be checked (ADA).

Forty to forty-nine years old

➤ Patients should review the guidelines for twenty- to thirty-nine-year-olds.

➤ Women age forty and older should get mammograms with (ACS) or without breast examination every one to two years (USPSTF).

➤ Patients forty-five years or older, especially those with a body mass index of 25 or greater, should consider getting tested for diabetes (ADA).

Fifty years old and older

➤ Patients should review the guidelines for twenty- to thirty-nine-year-olds and forty- to forty-nine-year-olds.

➤ Patients should be screened for colon cancer using either flexible sigmoidoscopy every five years with stool testing annually or colonoscopy every ten years or barium enema every ten years (USPSTF, ACS).

➤ Women sixty-five years and older should be routinely screened for osteoporosis. Those at high risk should be screened at age sixty (USPSTF).

➤ Men aged sixty-five to seventy-five years old who have smoked 100 or more cigarettes should have a one-time screening with ultrasound for abdominal aortic aneurysm (USPSTF).

DENIED COVERAGE? REIMBURSEMENT LETTER

In the event that the costs for your screening tests were denied by an insurance company, and assuming the costs are high enough that it is worth pursuing, begin by contacting the insurance company to seek an explanation of why routine tests are not considered a covered benefit. Write down the names of everyone you speak to, including the dates and times. Be sure to mention the following:

➤ The test in question (i.e. mammogram, colonoscopy, etc). When it was performed and by whom.

➤ The organization that recommends the test (i.e. American Cancer Society).

➤ The reason for the test (screening for breast cancer or colon cancer, for example).

➤ What you would like done (reimbursement for the co-pay, partial reimbursement, or full reimbursement).

If you do not receive a satisfactory answer, begin writing letters, always keeping a copy for yourself. To make sure the insurance company receives your letter, send them with a return receipt request. In the letter, again cover the facts as outlined above in addition to the names, dates, and times you spoke to their representatives. If that fails, contact your state government's insurance department for assistance.

TAKE-HOME POINTS

✓ *Life happens. Disease happens.* Wise patients get age- and gender-appropriate screening tests even if they feel healthy. They actively search for good health to make the most of their lives.

✓ *Consider getting immunized.*

✓ *Review the various guidelines* from the American Cancer Society, the American Heart Association, the American Diabetes Association, and the U. S. Preventive Services Task Force to see what tests you need to stay healthy.

PART FOUR:

Meet Your Medical Team

Doctor: one skilled or specializing in healing arts.
Derived from the Latin word *docere*, to teach.

— *Merriam-Webster's*

"Within the United States, adults with a primary care physician rather than a specialist had 33 percent lower cost of care and were 19 percent less likely to die, after adjusting for demographic and health characteristics"[88].

— *State of the Nation's Health Care 2007,*
The American College of Physicians, January 22, 2007

YOUR HEALTH ADVISORS: PHYSICIANS

Besides yourself, the most important person to keeping you healthy is your doctor. For many Americans, the primary care physician (PCP) or primary medical doctor (PMD) is the first logical entry point into the healthcare system and sometimes, particularly in rural areas, is the only physician they ever see for medical care. A highly trained and well-qualified primary care physician can advise you on what treatments and tests you truly need to stay healthy.

Primary care doctors are not all the same. Their level of training and scope of practice, as well as the issues they are able to handle, varies widely. Family medicine doctors, pediatricians, internists, and

> *A highly trained and well-qualified primary care physician can advise you on what treatments and tests you truly need to stay healthy.*

obstetrician/gynecologists (OB/Gyns) are traditionally considered primary care physicians. Family medicine physicians have the broadest scope of practice, caring for newborns and grandparents alike. Pediatricians care for newborns, young children, and adolescents, usually up to age eighteen. Internists care for adults and geriatric patients. OB/Gyns care solely for women. Unlike the other three specialists they also perform surgeries such as C-sections, hysterectomies, and bladder lifts or suspension repairs.

A good primary care physician is your trusted healthcare advisor. If you are generally healthy, you may only see a primary care physician your entire life. If you require more advanced or specialized medical care, your doctor can refer you to the right specialist. If you need many specialists, your doctor can help coordinate their care.

A good primary care doctor is an advocate for you. He gets feedback, advice, and information from all of your specialists to ensure that their care is in sync. Specialists often seem to work in a vacuum, focused exclusively on their field. To ensure that all of them are on the same page, it may be helpful to have one person oversee the overall treatment plan to maximize the benefit and minimize duplication of tests and procedures. Usually the primary care physician knows the patient the best and sees the individual as a person rather than a set of specific organ systems. As a result, you should receive better care.

Unfortunately, with the adoption of managed care in the 1990s, the term *primary care physician* began to be viewed negatively. The term became interchangeable with "gatekeeper." Patients saw gatekeepers as restricting or denying care. Patients were required to see their regular doctor to get a referral to see a specialist and prior authorization or approval for prescription medications not on the insurance plan's preferred list. In addition, during that time, insurance companies increased oversight on the doctors' use of tests, procedures, and medications and provided incentives to primary care doctors to minimize referrals. Though over time restrictions have lessened, and managed care has grown less common, these negative experiences still linger in the minds of both patients and physicians.

If there is to be one lesson learned from managed care, it is the value of having a primary care doctor as the first entry point into the healthcare system. *Primary care physicians can decrease costs and the amount of time wasted getting to the right specialists.* One health plan that focused on using primary care physicians to coordinate care discovered that use of specialists fell by 14 percent, emergency room use decreased by 16 percent, and prescriptions declined by 11 percent. When patients self-referred to specialists, about 60 percent went to the wrong specialist. This resulted in wasted time and money. On average, $1,500 was spent on various tests and diagnostic services visits over an eleven-month period before patients were told that the specialist could not help them. Clearly there is value in having a person help guide patients to the right place for care.

Although finding a good primary care doctor can be difficult today, in the future it may be even more so. Fewer medical students are choosing the fields of internal medicine and family medicine. This is largely because medical school is extremely expensive, and internists and family practitioners earn relatively little (and their salaries are decreasing)

One health plan that focused on using primary care physicians to coordinate care discovered that use of specialists fell by 14 percent, emergency room use decreased by 16 percent, and prescriptions declined by 11 percent. When patients self-referred to specialists, about 60 percent went to the wrong specialist.

compared to specialists. There is also the added complexity and uncertainly of caring for patients with complex medical histories. Only 19 percent of first-year resident physicians plan on practicing general internal medicine upon completion of their training program.[89] The remainder presumably will choose to go on to fellowship programs and specialize. Of those about to complete the three-year residency program in 2003, only 27 percent planned to be internists, down sharply from 54 percent in 1998.[90]

Others in practice are looking to avoid increasing overhead office costs, hassles from insurance companies, and decreasing reimbursement. About 35 percent of physicians are over the age of fifty-five, with most planning to retire over the next five to ten years.[91]

With current physicians planning on retiring soon and fewer replacing them, unless there are fundamental changes in the training and compensation of these fields, fewer U.S.-trained medical students will enter this field. As more baby boomers age and require additional medical care, there will be fewer primary care doctors available despite the increase in demand for their services. It's expected that in 2020 the nation will need about 147,000 internists, up 38 percent from 106,000 in 2000.[92] As the American College of Physicians said in 2006, "Without primary care, the healthcare system will become increasingly fragmented, over-specialized, and inefficient — leading to poorer quality care at higher costs."[93]

In a world where health care costs continue to increase and patients are shouldering more of the expenses, it's vital that you have a primary care physician. Wise patients always have a primary care physician. For adults, this should be either an internist or a family physician. Without one, it is very likely you will spend more and be less healthy.

Check Out Your Doctor Before He Checks You Out

Before your doctor's visit, figure out who you are dealing with. Many patients feel that their doctors are good if they can listen and communicate effectively, provide medical care easily and in a timely manner, and if patients have adequate control in making medical decisions.[94] While all doctors should have these abilities, these qualities alone do not necessarily mean the doctor is of high quality.

Even though he wears a white coat and carries a stethoscope and a title, what you really want to know is whether your doctor is licensed to practice in the state you live in, whether he is board certified, and other information that you might find helpful. You can easily find out these things on the Internet.

Importance of Board Certification

Your physician should be board certified in his field of expertise. To carry this distinction, your doctor must have graduated from an accredited residency program as well as passed the certification examination. The examination may be a one-day or two-day written test. Depending on the medical specialty, test takers may also need to take an oral examination.

Your physician should be board certified in his field of expertise.

To maintain their board certification, physicians are required to devote a certain number of hours per year to additional medical education. Doctors often fulfill this requirement by attending conferences and seminars. In addition, doctors must re-certify with a repeat examination every few years to continue their status. Given all of these requirements, a board-certified doctor will often provide the most up-to-date medical care. Ensure that your doctor is board certified.

Your physician may display his board certificate in the office. Some certificates may not have an expiration date because in the past, physicians only needed to take the exam once. It was good for life. This is no longer true. Current graduates can expect to retake the exam every seven to ten years.

Note that not all physicians who qualify to sit for the exam actually take it. Some providers in your insurance plan may not be board certified. The pass rate for first-time test takers varies anywhere from 84 percent to 94 percent.[95] You should only seek care with physicians who are board certified.

Licensing

Although your physician does not need to be board certified to practice medicine, he does need to be licensed. Find your own state medical board by going to the Federation of State Medical Boards at www.fsmb.org.

Each state provides different public information about its doctors. This typically includes the name of the physician, his license number, when the license was issued, and when it expires. Other states provide additional information like history of malpractice suits, felony convictions, or disciplinary action by the medical board. Some states split up the licensing and disciplinary functions into two different departments or websites. While at the state website, look for a link either for physician profile or credential search.

Training

Years ago it was possible for a medical school graduate to train an additional year through an internship, and then be able to set up an office practice as a general practitioner. But this is no longer the norm.

Today, an average graduate trains an additional three to five years in a residency program. Residency programs are where new doctors develop, hone, and refine their skills. Family medicine, pediatrics, and internal medicine require three years to complete the program. Obstetrics and gynecology takes four years. General surgery requires five years. The terms *intern* (first year resident), *resident* (second year or higher), and *chief resident* (the most senior resident) only occur in residency programs.

For certain specialties, even further advanced training is required. Fellowships can add another one to five years on top of the time spent in a residency. Fields of medicine that typically require fellowships include cardiology (heart — cardiovascular system), endocrinology (thyroid, diabetes), pulmonology (lung — respiratory system), rheumatology (muscles, joints), hematology/oncology (diseases of the blood/cancer), infectious diseases, nephrology (kidneys), and gastroenterology (stomach, colon, liver). Allergists and immunologists need to be board certified in either internal medicine or pediatrics prior to doing their fellowship.

There are also surgical fellowships. These include but are not limited to breast surgery, colon and rectal surgery, pediatric surgery, plastic surgery, transplants, and vascular surgery. In total there are over 140 different fields one can train in.[96]

Why is this important to know? Because each of these fields has an accrediting board which set standards of care. Physicians who are board certified graduated from an accredited residency and/or fellowship program and passed the governing board's certification exam. Think of it as the difference between hiring a certified public accountant (CPA) and someone who just files taxes for you. While you might get the same result, if difficult issues come up, you may not get the best advice.

Residency programs and fellowships can be based at public county hospitals, private community hospitals, or tertiary university medical centers. The education and experience physicians get vary. Physicians at a public county hospital often see people with common diseases like diabetes, heart disease, and high blood pressure. Most of these patients are indigent, do not have health insurance, and do not get preventive care. Their illnesses often lead to serious complications not commonly seen in the general community.

Physicians who train at these facilities are very familiar with treating these illnesses and complications and have a wealth of hands-on experience.

Doctors who train at tertiary medical centers — for example, university hospitals — may have a completely different experience. Community physicians frequently refer patients with rare illnesses or complex medical problems to academic medical centers, which often have greater resources and expertise. Since the university hospital becomes a magnet for these cases, these doctors see many patients with unusual illnesses that a practicing physician might see only once in an entire career. Physicians studying to become specialists benefit most from this arrangement as they get the opportunity to treat common problems, but also experience a large number of rare or difficult cases.

In general, however, physicians from either of these types of programs are well trained.

INTERNISTS AND FAMILY PHYSICIANS

Although the terms sound similar, internists and family physicians are very different doctors. Internists, or internal medicine physicians, spend their three years of residency focused solely on adult care. The residency is often based in a hospital, where residents care for patients in the intensive care units, telemetry (heart monitored) units, and general medical floors. There, a patient's care may be managed completely by the internist or in conjunction with a team of specialists, depending on the situation.

Internists also train outside the hospital, working in the emergency room and other outpatient (office) settings. Some of their time is spent with spe-

> *Although the terms sound similar, internists and family physicians are very different doctors.*

cialists from cardiology, rheumatology, nephrology, and others to provide these physicians with a well-rounded education.

With experience caring for hospitalized patients, as well as knowledge grounded in general medicine and supplemented with specialty education, graduates can begin practicing as internists. Some, however, may decide to enroll in a fellowship program to exclusively focus on a medical specialty like cardiology, nephrology, or gastroenterology. Depending on the field, this training adds two to five years to their general medicine residency. Certification is overseen by the American Board of Internal Medicine (ABIM) www.abim.org.

Although family physicians also have a three-year residency program, their training focuses on caring for all patients in all age groups, from newborns to geriatrics, and includes some obstetrics. The bulk of family physicians' training is in the office setting, caring for babies, children, adolescents, adults, pregnant women, and seniors. Some training also takes place in the hospital. Graduates can undergo additional training and add certification in sports, adolescent, and/or geriatric medicine.

One of the distinguishing features of family medicine is its view of the patient as a whole, which includes looking at how the family and other factors impact a patient's health. To better understand this perspective, resident physicians often train with psychologists. The American Board of Family Medicine (ABFM) is responsible for board certification. A physician's standing can be verified at www.theabfm.org.

A generalist, general practitioner, or GP is not exactly the same as a family physician. A GP is a medical school graduate who only finished one year of residency (i.e., did an internship) and went on to practice medicine. Fewer graduates today are GPs, as most opt to complete a full residency program.

Depending on the individual physician's training, graduates from either an internal medicine or family medicine residency program might

Adults should always have a board-certified internist or a family physician as their primary care doctor.

be comfortable with and knowledgeable about office procedures like skin biopsies, ingrown toenail removals, injection of joints with cortisone, insertion of IUDs (intrauterine devices), Pap smears, flexible sigmoidoscopies, interpreting cardiac stress tests (treadmill test), or placing stitches. The only way you know is to ask.

The kind of physician you seek often depends on where you live. If you live in a rural community where there are only a handful of physicians, your primary care physician probably does a lot more procedures both in scope and number than his counterpart, who practices in a large suburban setting where specialists are easily available. With more physicians available to you in a larger city, you may prefer to see a specialist even though your regular physician can provide the same services.

Also, consider whether your primary care physician can perform these tests and procedures at the level of a specialist. If you aren't sure or comfortable, ask your doctor or go see a specialist. Physicians who are competent and confident should not be offended by this question. Asking can seem intimidating, but remember it is your health.

Besides typical medical procedures, many physicians provide additional services due to decreasing reimbursements. Doctors can enroll in weekend/weeklong conferences to learn skills like botox injections and laser skin treatment for removal of tattoos and wrinkles to improve their revenues. These procedures can be performed during an office visit. Whether you want your doctor to perform these procedures is entirely up to you.

Adults should always have a board-certified internist or a family physician as their primary care doctor.

SPECIALISTS

There may be times when you or your physician decides that consulting a specialist is necessary. Specialists are highly trained in a specific field, either on a particular organ or organ system (the cardiologist is focused on the heart and cardiovascular system, while a neurologist is focused on the nervous system) or a disease process (an oncologist treats cancer; an infectious disease specialist manages infections). Surgical specialists' niche is similarly focused on a particular organ system or skill within the surgical field (a vascular surgeon performs blood vessel bypass, for example).

Specialists' training requirements vary depending on the specialty. Most applicants are required to have completed a full three-year residency in internal medicine before entering a fellowship program in the medical specialties. Other specialty fields, like radiology and psychiatry, require applicants to complete a one-year internship, known as a transitional year, before joining a specific residency program. The transitional year is usually spent in an internal medicine residency program.

Much like medical specialties, surgical subspecialties may require applicants to have completed a general residency program prior to beginning their fellowship training. A general surgery residency usually is five years.

Verify whether your specialist is board certified in his area of expertise by going to the American Board of Medical Specialties at www. abms.org. Click on the Member Boards link. Also refer to www.abim.org, the website for the American Board of Internal Medicine (ABIM).

Make the most of your visit by understanding what each of these specialists has to offer. The following list identifies specialists commonly utilized by

Make the most of your visit by understanding what each of these specialists has to offer.

a primary care physician and procedures and skills that patients may need or encounter. For simplicity this list is divided into medical and surgical specialties.

MEDICAL SPECIALTIES

Who: Allergist/Immunologist

What: Evaluates, diagnoses, and treats conditions like asthma; skin conditions like eczema and urticaria (hives); allergies due to environmental factors, medications, foods, and insects; and immune system problems.

Special Tests/Procedures: skin testing, allergy shots, and lung testing.

Training: Two-year fellowship program after completing either a pediatric or an internal medicine three-year residency program.

More Info: American Academy of Allergy Asthma and Immunology, www.aaaai.org. American College of Allergy, Asthma, and Immunology, www.acaai.org.

Who: Cardiologist

What: Diagnoses and treats conditions of the heart and circulatory system (like the arteries), including hypertension (high blood pressure), myocardial infarctions (heart attacks), angina or coronary artery disease (heart disease), arrhythmias (irregular heart beats), heart valve problems, and other diseases. You might see a cardiologist if your heart problem cannot be adequately treated, managed, or evaluated by your regular doctor.

Special Tests/Procedures: Electrocardiogram (EKG), treadmill stress test (a treadmill hooked up to a heart monitor), or echocardiogram (ultrasound of the heart). Interventional cardiologists, a subset of cardiologists, require additional training and can perform cardiac catheterizations and placement of stents or pacemakers. These procedures are done in a catheter lab which is usually part of a hospital or ambulatory surgery center. Cardiologists do not perform open heart surgery.

Training: A two- to four-year fellowship program.

More Info: The American College of Cardiology, www.acc.org.

Who: Dermatologist

What: Diagnoses and treats skin conditions like acne, dermatitis, psoriasis; skin cancers like basal cell cancer, squamous cell cancer, and melanoma; or abnormalities of the hair and nails. You might see a dermatologist if you have a stubborn rash or dermatitis that does not get better or an abnormal spot that does not go away.

Special Tests/Procedures: Treatments can include light therapy (photo therapy) and/or medications like creams, pills, and now in some cases intravenous therapies (IV), depending on the condition. Procedures include removal of moles or skin cancers with biopsy, freezing the area with liquid nitrogen, destroying it with cautery, or scraping the area with a curette.

Training: A total of four years, with the first year as a transitional year and the last three in a dermatology residency program. Graduates can receive fellowship training in cosmetic dermatology, pediatric dermatology, dermatopathology (more specialized than general pathology), Mohs surgery (a surgical technique that allows removal of skin cancers in delicate areas of the face like the nose and ears), and others.

More Info: The American Academy of Dermatology, www.aad.org.

Who: **Endocrinologist**

What: Evaluates and treats conditions related to the endocrine system which can include the thyroid, pancreas, and pituitary and adrenal glands. Typical problems include diabetes and thyroid conditions, among many others.

Special Tests/Procedures: thyroid biopsy.

Training: Two-year fellowship after a three-year internal medicine residency program.

More Info: The Endocrine Society at www.endo-society.org.

Who: **Gastroenterologist**

What: Diagnoses and treats conditions of the digestive system beginning at the esophagus and ending at the rectum. Problems include heartburn; cancers of the esophagus, stomach, and colon; irritable bowel syndrome; inflammatory bowel disease (ulcerative colitis and Crohn's disease); liver cirrhosis; and hepatitis, to name a few. Oral prescription medications as well as intravenous medications are used depending on the problem.

Special Tests/Procedures: Esophagogastroduodenoscopy (EGD — also known as an upper endoscopy) to evaluate the esophagus, stomach, and duodenum and a colonoscopy to check the large intestine. Dilation of the esophagus can be done if there is scar tissue causing a problem with swallowing food. Placement of a permanent feeding tube is also done with an EGD. Both the EGD and colonoscopy procedures are performed with a patient sedated by IV medications and are used to diagnose, screen, and/or monitor for cancer. Flexible sigmoidoscopy is used to evaluate the large intestine.

Training: A two- to three-year fellowship program.

More Info: The American College of Gastroenterology has a patient friendly website at www.acg.gi.org.

Who: Hematologist/Oncologist — also known as "Hem/Onc."

What: Diagnoses and evaluates problems with the blood system which includes the red blood cells, white blood cells, bone marrow, platelets, and coagulation system. Oncologists diagnose and treat various types of cancers including breast, colon, lung, ovarian, pancreatic, stomach, lymphoma, leukemia, and many others. Treatments can involve use of powerful medications known as chemotherapy, in addition to arranging other options like radiation therapy and biologic therapy (like using specific target therapies tailored to an individual patient's cancer).

Special Tests/Procedures: Office procedures include a bone marrow biopsy where a needle is inserted into the bone (typically the hip) to analyze the health of the bone marrow and intrathecal injections where medications are placed into the fluid surrounding the brain.

Training: A three-year fellowship program. Typically hematology and oncology training is combined, hence the phrase "hem/onc."

More Info: The American Society of Hematology has a website with a patient section at www.hematology.org. The American Society of Clinical Oncology (ASCO) website is www.asco.org. It also supports a good website for cancer patients at www.peoplelivingwithcancer.org.

Who: Nephrologist

What: Focuses on diseases and problems of the kidney. Prevents kidney failure and deteriorating kidney function as well as maintains and/or improves kidney function with prescription medications and patient counseling about kidney-safe diets and medications. Uses dialysis machines, which process the blood, clean it of toxins, and balance the electrolytes, for patients suffering from kidney failure.

Special Tests/Procedures: Kidney biopsy, the placement of an
     intravenous central line that can be used temporarily for
     dialysis.

Training: Two-year fellowship program.

More Info: www.asn-online.org.

Who: **Neurologist**

What: Diagnoses and treats conditions that affect the nervous
     system (the brain, spinal cord, and other nerves). Conditions
     can include migraine headaches, multiple sclerosis, strokes,
     Alzheimer's, dementia, and seizures.

Special Tests/Procedures: Lumbar puncture (a needle inserted in
     the low back to evaluate the spinal fluid), nerve conduction
     test (electrodes placed into nerves to check functioning), and
     EEGs (electrodes attached to the scalp to measure brain wave
     activity and often used in the evaluation of seizures).

Training: A three-year residency program after completion of a
     transitional year.

More Info: The American Academy of Neurology website is
     www.aan.com.

Who: **Pulmonologist**

What: Diagnoses and treats conditions related to the respiratory
     system. This can include asthma, emphysema or COPD (chronic
     obstructive pulmonary disease), cystic fibrosis, and sleep
     apnea. Treatments include inhaled prescription medications,
     oral pills, and/or use of oxygen. Manages patients on
     ventilators.

Special Tests/Procedures: Pulmonary function test (PFT)
     — determines an individual's lung capacity and function.
     Bronchoscopy is using a thin flexible tube with a fiber optic

camera to evaluate the trachea (windpipe) and smaller airways (bronchi and bronchioles). Thoracentesis is using a needle to remove fluid from the lungs. In the situation of a collapsed lung, a chest tube can be placed in the chest area to re-expand the lung.

Training: A two-year fellowship program. Graduates can receive additional training in critical care medicine (treatment of critically ill patients in the intensive care unit) or pediatric pulmonology.

More Info: American College of Chest Physicians, www.chestnet.org.

Who: Rheumatologist

What: Diagnoses and treats diseases like osteoarthritis (the arthritis most common among older patients), rheumatoid arthritis, lupus, fibromyalgia, gout, and vasculitis. Evaluates patients with muscle or joint achiness and swelling, especially when there was no overuse or injury, which can be caused by systemic illness. (Injured joints are often seen by an orthopedist.)

Special Tests/Procedures: Injection of the joints with medications like cortisone, removing fluid from joints for evaluation. The use of intravenous (IV) medications to treat inflammatory conditions like rheumatoid arthritis. Rheumatologists do not operate or perform surgery.

Training: A two-year fellowship program.

More Info: The American College of Rheumatology has a good website for the public at www.rheumatology.org.

SURGICAL SPECIALTIES

Who: **General Surgeon**

What: Performs appendectomies, gallbladder surgery, repair/removal of varicose veins, hemorrhoids, and growth/tumor removal from the breast or other parts of the body. Generally focuses on surgery in the abdominal area as well as breast, but depending on the training some also operate around the neck (thyroid) and other areas typically covered by surgical subspecialists.

Special Tests/Procedures: Aside from surgeries in the operating room, office-based biopsies and procedures. May do sigmoidoscopies prior to hemorrhoid surgery.

Training: A five-year residency program.

More Info: American College of Surgeons, www.facs.org.

Who: **Ophthalmologist**

What: Treats all diseases of the eye. Not to be confused with optometrists, who deal mainly with determining and fitting patients with corrective lenses, glasses, or contact lenses.

Special Tests/Procedures: Eye surgery for cataracts, glaucoma, and retinal detachments, as well as corrective surgeries.

Training: A one-year transitional program followed by a three- to four-year ophthalmology residency program.

More Info: American Academy of Ophthalmology, www.aao.org.

Who: **Orthopedist**

What: Treats problems of the bones and muscles including arthritis, fractures, and muscle pulls and strains. These problems are typically due to mechanical causes like overuse or physical injury. Unlike rheumatologists, orthopedists operate on joints to repair, rehabilitate, or replace.

Special Tests/Procedures: Cortisone injections in joints like the elbow, shoulder, knee, wrist, and hip. Joint replacement (knee or hip).

Training: Five-year residency program. Fellowships include musculoskeletal oncology (the treatment of bone and muscle cancers), sports medicine, and shoulder and knee programs.

More Info: Learn more at the American Academy of Orthopaedic Surgeons at www.aaos.org.

Who: Otolaryngologist

What: Treats diseases and problems of the ears, nose, throat, sinuses, and neck.

Special Tests/Procedures: Examination of the nasal passages, sinuses, throat, and vocal cords with a small thin flexible tube known as a nasopharyngoscope. Surgeries can include placement of ear tubes, sinus surgery, palate repair, and biopsy and surgical removal of head and neck cancers.

Training: One transitional year in general surgery and four years of specialty surgery.

More Info: American Board of Otolaryngology at www.aboto.org.

OTHER PRIMARY CARE FIELDS

Who: Obstetrician/Gynecologist

What: Cares for women and treats conditions and disorders of the female reproductive and urinary tract. Provides care to pregnant women and delivers babies.

Special Tests/Procedures: Pelvic surgeries, including hysterectomies and tubal ligations. Pap smear to screen for cervical cancer and a colposcopy to detect and treat early cervical cancer. Ultrasound to evaluate a fetus. Cesarean section or vaginal delivery of a baby.

Training: Four-year residency program. Additional fellowships can be done in maternal fetal medicine, which focuses on the management of high-risk pregnancies; gynecology/oncology, the surgical treatment of reproductive cancers; and urogynecology, the treatment of urinary tract disorders.

More Info: American College of Obstetricians and Gynecologists, www.acog.org.

Who: **Pediatrician**

What: Cares for newborns, toddlers, children, teenagers, and young adults.

Special Tests/Procedures: Evaluates the development of children and treats illnesses and problems that affect them.

Training: Three-year residency program. Fellowships can be done in neonatal medicine, the treatment of premature and newborn babies, as well as other specialties like endocrinology, hematology/oncology, infectious disease, nephrology, neurology, and others.

More info: American Academy of Pediatrics, www.aap.org.

OTHER SPECIALTIES

Who: **Emergency Medicine Physicians**

What: Treats acute and/or potentially life threatening problems of patients in the emergency room.

Special Tests/Procedures: Lumbar puncture, minor surgeries and laceration repair, casting of broken bones, placement of chest tubes, endotracheal tubes (to attach to a ventilator), and many others.

Training: A three-year residency program after a one-year transitional program.

More Info: American College of Emergency Physicians, www.acep.org.

Who: **Psychiatrist**

What: Treats cognitive, mental, or emotional disorders like anxiety, depression, bipolar disorder, schizophrenia, eating disorders, phobias, and many others. Prescribes medications for various illnesses.

Special Tests/Procedures: Supervises electroconvulsive therapy (ECT), shock treatment for severely depressed patients.

Training: A three-year residency program after a one-year transitional program. Additional fellowship training can be done in geriatric psychiatry, child and adolescent psychiatry, or addiction medicine.

More Info: www.healthyminds.org; www.psych.org.

WHAT'S THE DEAL WITH DOs (DOCTORS OF OSTEOPATHIC MEDICINE)?

MDs are also known as doctors of allopathic medicine. Some doctors aren't MDs at all; they're DOs, or doctors of osteopathic medicine. The DO field started in 1874 in America, when Dr. Andrew Taylor Still focused less on medications and more on keeping the whole body, particularly the musculoskeletal system, healthy.[97]

This belief is reflected in DOs' training. Like MDs, DOs typically complete four years of undergraduate study and four years of medical training. Although osteopathic medical schools have a similar curriculum to allopathic medical school, students receive additional training on the musculoskeletal system and osteopathic manipulative treatment (OMT). This latter skill allows DOs to use their hands to diagnose illness and stimulate the body to recover.

After graduation, more than half of all DOs go on to residency training programs in primary care fields like pediatrics, OB/GYN, internal medicine, and family medicine. As a patient, you might not

Some doctors use other medical providers, known as physician extenders, to help them provide direct patient care. These are physician assistants and nurse practitioners.

notice any difference between your DO and your MD, and you should still address your DO as doctor. Nevertheless, DOs are considered a separate branch of medicine and they do take comparable but different state licensing exams. Some states, like Arizona, California, and Michigan, have set up separate agencies to regulate licensure and oversee the practice of DOs than those that govern MDs.

OTHER PROVIDERS

Some doctors use other medical providers, known as *physician extenders,* to help them provide direct patient care. These are physician assistants and nurse practitioners. Unlike support staff, these physician extenders may be the ones directly taking care of you.

Physician Assistants (PAs)

According to the American Academy of Physician Assistants website, www.aapa.org, the concept of a physician assistant (PA) started in the 1960s when physicians and educators noted that there were an inadequate number of primary care physicians.[98] PAs are licensed to practice medicine while under the supervision of a physician.

PA training programs are much shorter than those for physicians. Most PA training programs last two years and require that applicants have had least two years of college and some experience in the health care field. In 2005, there were approximately 55,000 practicing PAs. They are allowed to write prescriptions (except in Indiana and Ohio).

Physician assistants certified by the National Commission on Certification have the title of PA-C. To maintain this standing, they are required to take a recertification examination every six years and complete a total of one hundred hours of continuing education every two years.

The American Medical Association has recommended some guidelines about how physicians and PAs should interact with each other. An important one for all patients to be aware of is this:

> Patients should be made clearly aware at all times whether they are being cared for by a physician or a physician assistant.

Patients should be made clearly aware at all times whether they are being cared for by a physician or a physician assistant.

Therefore, you should always ask who is treating you. Since PAs are not physicians, their title is usually Mr. or Ms. If you are not sure, ask. In medical school we had an occasional physician assistant student with us when we were working in the hospital. With our short white coats, stethoscopes, and eager faces, I know our patients did not realize which students were becoming MDs and which were training to be PAs.

For common medical problems, PAs are usually adequate. However, *if you are not comfortable with seeing a PA, ask and even demand to see a physician. It is your health and your money.* Good PAs know their limits, and depending on the situation will actually recommend you see their physician supervisor. Bad PAs think they're doctors and don't know their limits. If your condition is not improving under the care of a PA, consider seeing a doctor.

Nurse Practitioners (NPs)

The American Academy of Nurse Practitioners, www.aanp.org, represents over 85,000 practicing nurse practitioners.[99] Prior to becoming an NP, the vast majority of applicants have masters' degrees in nursing.

Roughly 80 percent of NPs are in the field of family medicine or adult medicine. Those who have completed a master's-level training program can sit for certification examinations in these fields and can use the title of NP-C. Recertification is done every five years and requires either retaking the examination or showing proof of at least one thousand hours of clinical practice and seventy-five hours of continuing education in the relevant field of practice.

OFFICE SETTINGS

Most of the time your care is delivered in an office setting but the options vary. You could see your doctor in a private practice office, at an academic medical center, or at an integrated healthcare system. While all settings provide good care, it is your preference that matters, as your experience in each one will be different.

Private Practice

Many patients are familiar with the private practice office. In the past, it was the main option for most physicians who wanted to "hang their own shingle" and begin a successful career. The doctor who owns the practice has complete authority over managing the office, ranging from selection of office space and furniture to choosing staff and equipment to determining office hours and which insurance plans to accept. These doctors are true entrepreneurs.

The number of physicians in an office can range from a sole practitioner and one receptionist/nurse to a group of physicians from different specialties and their support staff all under one roof.

Because physicians in this setting are self-employed, should you have concerns about the staff or the care you receive, you can ask to speak to the boss. He or she will usually be a doctor. This doctor has an incentive to keep you happy and retain you as a patient.

Pharmaceutical representatives are sometimes also around in this setting. They may be waiting in the lobby or in the back educating doctors on their latest medications and supplying free medication samples. They may also feed the office staff with lunch. You can spot them easily as they are professionally dressed in business suits, often cart around a small box of medication samples or pens, and are requesting signatures from the physician to indicate receipt of the medication samples. They may appear hurried as they move on quickly to the next doctor's office.

Although it's hard to believe, given how much we pay for health care, insurance reimbursements to physicians have been declining relative to inflation. As a result, physicians are trying to see more patients per day to recoup some of their income. Others doctors, in an effort to improve income, are offering services like botox injections and laser treatment of tattoos and skin spots to cash-paying patients. It is not easy, financially, to be in private practice. This means, sadly, that the trend of rushed physicians or those providing additional services for a fee will not go away.

Residency Training Programs/Academic Medical Centers

Patients who choose to get care at a residency training program or an academic medical center often have a rewarding experience. Your "doctor" can be a medical student, a resident physician, or an attending physician, who supervises the previous two doctors in training and is the physician of record. The focus of these programs is not only to provide you with good care, but also to teach new physicians how to do just that. If you have an uncommon disease, symptom, or unique physical trait, don't be surprised if you find yourself surrounded by a group of inquisitive medical students and residents. Most of these patients often joke that they would be quite rich if they charged a couple of dollars for each viewing.

The advantage of academic medical centers is that you may be receiving the most up-to-date care. Medical students and resident physicians focus not only on the basics of medicine but also routinely review and critique the latest research studies as part of their training. They often spend more time asking detailed questions about your illnesses and performing a thorough physical exam than more experienced doctors. The other advantage is that you are helping new physicians learn their craft, and could positively influence them as physicians.

The downside of an academic medical center is that you might spend more time in the office. Medical students and interns do not have medical licenses and need to discuss your case with their attending physician. Depending on the experience of your "doctor," the severity of the problem, and the familiarity of the attending physician with your provider, you may be questioned and examined again by the supervising physician. Don't worry. You are not a guinea pig. Think of it more as an apprenticeship. Ultimately, your health and care are the responsibility of the licensed attending physician. This entire process, however, can be time consuming.

Another problem is that you might not be able to see the same person over a period of time. Doctors in training change their clinical rotations every few weeks and new doctors come in to take their place. Even if you manage to see your doctor for an extended period of time, they all inevitably graduate and move on to begin their careers.

Integrated Healthcare Offices

You may find this kind of setting at a large integrated HMO system, at the Veterans Administration (VA) hospitals, or academic medical centers, all of which hire physicians as staff. Unlike in private practice offices, physicians who work in integrated healthcare offices are salaried employees. Because they are not in charge, they have little influence over office hours, staff, furniture, or the equipment they use. And because these providers are salaried, they may not have a financial incentive to see many patients. However, these physicians *are* accountable to their employers, who may have productivity goals or other responsibilities that must be fulfilled.

The advantage of an integrated system is that communication and medical information can potentially flow more easily between the different doctors involved in your care. A system that contains patient records, medications, and test results through one common database makes it easier for physicians to collaborate with one another to provide care. An integrated system can be more efficient, because doctors of different specialties don't duplicate efforts. In fact, studies suggest that this kind of system might deliver better care than the traditional fragmented system where community doctors practice independently.

Studies suggest that this kind of system might deliver better care than the traditional fragmented system where community doctors practice independently.

The VA healthcare system, for example, provides better care on many quality measures like screenings for cancer, diabetic blood sugar control, and appropriate use of medications, compared to the care delivered by local providers to their patients with private insurance. The VA also outscored its local counterparts in patient satisfaction surveys.[100] Similarly, the integrated healthcare system Kaiser Permanente has been identified by federal officials, healthcare economists, and other external organizations as a group that delivers better care. Patients in the Northern California Kaiser Permanente program have a 30 percent lower death rate from heart disease than identically matched patients in the rest of the community.[101]

TAKE-HOME POINTS

✓ Wise patients always have a primary care doctor. For adults, a primary care doctor is either an internist or a family physician.

✓ Before seeing a doctor, do some research. Your physician should be board certified in his field of practice. Find out at www.abms.org.

✓ At times you may require the expertise of a specialist. Make the most of your visit by understanding what special knowledge, skills, and treatments the specialist can offer you and why you are going.

✓ Other providers, like physician assistants (PAs) or nurse practitioners (NPs), may be involved in your care. You should always be informed of this. If you prefer to see a physician, say so. It's your health and your money.

✓ Medical care can be received in three practice settings: the private office, an academic medical center, or in an integrated healthcare system. Each environment has different benefits and tradeoffs. Find the one that works for you.

PART FIVE:

The Truth About Medications

> "One of the first duties of the physician is to educate the masses not to take medicine."[102]
>
> "The desire to take medicine is perhaps the greatest feature which distinguishes man from animals."
>
> — **Dr. William Osler, famous John Hopkins physician who transformed clinical teaching of physicians in the 1890s.**[103]

THE MAGIC PILLS

The Business of Marketing Medications

Health care has become more complicated since Dr. Osler uttered those statements over a century ago. Physicians today have many more medications at their disposal than Dr. Osler did. Medications help heal us (antibiotics); relieve troubling symptoms (antihistamines, steroid nasal sprays for allergies); or keep us healthy by preventing illness and complications (cholesterol-lowering medications, high blood pressure medications). Much of the improvement in life expectancy over the past century is due to advances in medication.

After health insurance premiums, medication costs are the second most significant healthcare expense.

Perhaps it is not surprising, then, that *after health insurance premiums, medication costs are the second most significant healthcare expense.* As employers and workers struggle with rising premiums, many others are equally concerned about their ability to pay for prescription drugs. Medication costs continue to rise faster than inflation and patients are responsible for more of the costs.

Trying to get by with less medication comes at a price. A study showed that patients with pre-existing health conditions who cut back on their prescriptions were 76 percent more likely to have worsened their health; 50 percent were more likely to have a non-fatal heart attack, stroke, or chest pain, and their health declined within two to three years.[104]

Medication costs are rising faster than other products and services for a variety of reasons. First, people are living longer with conditions like high cholesterol, high blood pressure, asthma, and diabetes. Consequently, for them to continue to stay healthy, they need to continue taking their medications. Second, Americans are less healthy than in the past. More young people are developing medical problems traditionally thought to be the domain of middle-aged patients. Understandably, as people live longer and more individuals are diagnosed with conditions that need treatment, more prescriptions will be dispensed. From 1997 to 2001, the number of prescriptions written increased by 29 percent, or from 2.4 billion in 1997 to 3.1 billion in 2001.

Another reason for the increase in cost is that physicians are prescribing more expensive medications. Of the over 9,500 medications available, just fifty accounted for a whopping 45 percent of total sales.[105] Only five of the 50 medications were the less costly generic variety. From 1997 to 2001, the total spent on prescriptions nearly doubled, from $78.9 billion in 1997 to 154.5 billion in 2001, clearly outpacing the 29 percent increase in volume.[106]

The question is whether newer and pricier medications are worth the added cost. For a new medication to get FDA approval, a manufacturer simply needs to show that it is better than a placebo. The manufacturer does not need to compare it to existing therapies or generic medications. If a company wishes to fund a head-to-head study of its new drug against comparable medications, it usually does so for other reasons besides FDA approval — to provide physicians proof that its product is superior, for example. Would it surprise you to discover that a company-sponsored study typically found its medication to be better?

Pharmaceutical companies heavily market newer and more expensive medications in order to create demand.

Pharmaceutical companies heavily market newer and more expensive medications in order to create demand. Take the example of the anti-inflammatory medication Vioxx, manufactured by Merck. Research studies showed that Vioxx was less likely to cause stomach ulcers or bleeding, side effects common to other medications in this class (like ibuprofen and naprosyn). Vioxx was marketed as being gentler on the stomach, while still providing pain relief similar to that of other anti-inflammatories. Of course, ulcers and bleeding are uncommon side effects in the first place, usually seen in older patients and those with previous histories of stomach problems.

Comparably effective but potentially safer for a small number of patients at high risk for stomach irritation, Vioxx should have been a niche product. Instead, it was marketed to everyone who needed pain relief. In 2000, Merck spent more money ($160 million) promoting Vioxx than PepsiCo spent marketing Pepsi ($120 million) or Anheuser-Busch spent on promoting Budweiser beer ($140 million). In fact, Vioxx was the most heavily advertised medication in 2000. Between 1999, when Vioxx was introduced, and 2000, sales skyrocketed from $329.5 million to $1.5 billion.[107]

Vioxx is only one of many examples of how patients are fooled into believing that newer advertised medications are better than older,

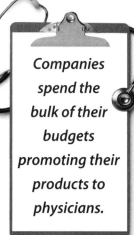

Companies spend the bulk of their budgets promoting their products to physicians.

less exciting medications when there is no scientific evidence to prove it. In the ads, people are encouraged to ask if a particular medication is "right for [them]." The commercials overstate the effectiveness of the product or minimize the side effects. In many instances, federal agencies have asked pharmaceutical companies to revise their advertisements because they were misleading.

Unfortunately, the general public isn't the only group that advertising targets. Companies spend the bulk of their budgets promoting their products to physicians. Of the $15 billion spent on marketing in 2000, 84 percent of that was spent educating physicians at the office (25 percent), in a hospital setting (5 percent), or in a magazine ad (3 percent). A little over 50 percent of the money was used to provide medication samples. By comparison, only 16 percent, or $2.5 billion, was used to advertise to consumers.[108] Companies continue to expand their marketing budgets and staff. In 1996, there was about one pharmaceutical representative for every eighteen physicians. Ten years later there is one for every nine.[109]

The relationship between pharmaceutical representatives and physicians starts early. Medical students receive free pens, mugs, and lunches. A 2005 article noted that on average a third-year medical student received one gift, or attended one program sponsored by a pharmaceutical company, per week.[110] Of the over eight hundred medical students surveyed, 68.8 percent said that they would not change their practice even with the gifts. Ironically, they felt less confident about their classmates' ability to stay unbiased. Only 57.7 percent felt that their colleagues would not be influenced.

When practicing physicians were asked in similar surveys about their objectivity when receiving gifts from pharmaceutical companies, the results mirrored those of the medical students. The majority felt that their colleagues and peers were less objective than they were.

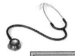 **Real-Life Example**

When I was a resident physician, I, like many of my colleagues, welcomed the opportunity to get a free dinner sponsored by a pharmaceutical representative. As residents, we worked long hours for little money. Any chance for free food was a no brainer: take it!

But we weren't the only ones in attendance. The representatives would often invite us at the last minute. Their main focus was on the practicing doctors in the community, who could write many more prescriptions than we could. Often these doctors would bring their spouses to these nice restaurants. During dinner, we listened to a presentation about a particular medication.

What surprised me is how fast and willing the doctors were to agree with the presenter. One evening, the discussion centered around a fairly new cholesterol-lowering medication. The presenter showed how the product lowered cholesterol much better than the competition. Conspicuously absent was any research that showed whether the medicine *saved lives*. While one can assume that lowering cholesterol would help prevent heart disease, without proof that statement is just an assumption.

Once the presentation was completed, the moderator asked each physician if he would consider prescribing this medication to his next patient. Everyone said yes. When it was my turn, I asked about the absence of research that proved this medication would save lives. Without it, I said,

I would be less likely to write a prescription.

The willingness to prescribe disappeared rather quickly as the remaining physicians also expressed their reservations. Perhaps the other colleagues thought the same but felt impolite about making a fuss. I don't know. But one thing is for certain: doctors are writing prescriptions for more expensive medications.

Times are changing, albeit very slowly. In 2005, a handful of medical centers, including those at the University of Pennsylvania, Yale, and Stanford, as well as the integrated healthcare organization Kaiser Permanente, began prohibiting their physicians from receiving gifts from pharmaceutical representatives.[111] This is a small step in the right direction.

So, as a patient, what can you do? First, be aware of the tremendous amount of money invested by companies to promote their medications to you, the consumer, and to your physicians. When you see an advertisement for a medication you can be sure that **one** of the following applies:

➤ It is brand new.

➤ It is an existing medication that has new FDA approval to be used for another illness or condition.

➤ It is not generic, and therefore likely expensive.

➤ It may have many competitors. The pharmaceutical company is trying to increase its sales, market share, and brand loyalty.

➤ It is a new version of an existing medication which is about to go off patent. The pharmaceutical company is trying to get patients to switch to the newer product, which will have patent protection.

It is unfortunate that medications are promoted the same way as other things we buy at
the grocery store. Patients can get coupons for
a discount or a free trial. Unlike toiletries and
household products, these items can cause serious side effects that can be dangerous. Instead of
requesting specific medications, ask your doctor
about a particular symptom or problem the advertisement prompted you to think about. Switching
medications, particularly ones that are heavily promoted, may not necessarily be better for you — but it
will likely be more expensive.

> *Switching medications, particularly ones that are heavily promoted, may not necessarily be better for you — but it will likely be more expensive.*

The burden of deciding which medication to use
is still ultimately up to your doctor. To minimize the
influence advertising has on your doctor, it's important
that you know the difference between generic and branded medications, what questions to ask your doctor, and when taking a branded
medication might be a good idea. Only then can you have an honest
discussion about prescription medications and be more comfortable
with the choices you will make with your physician.

GENERIC AND BRANDED MEDICATIONS: WHAT'S THE DIFFERENCE?

Most patients switch to generic medications to save money. They
often do so with great reluctance, though, as they wonder if they are simply taking an inferior product. A patient will ask himself, does changing
from a branded to a generic medication harm my health? Is switching
the right thing to do? No one likes to trade down for a cheaper, older
product, especially if the perception is that newer is better. Is there a
difference between generic and branded medications?

Patients usually don't change to generics because of more extensive safety and side effect information: they choose generics because *they typically cost only a fraction of branded medications.* Think of branded medications as similar to household names like Coke and Pepsi, while generics are the sodas sold by supermarkets and drug stores under their own name. The former are heavily marketed; the latter are usually much cheaper and aren't marketed at all. But they're both sugary and fizzy, and serve about the same purpose. While I suspect that there are some diehard Coke and Pepsi drinkers, for most of us these sodas are all about the same.

Generally, there is no significant difference between a generic medication and its branded counterpart. Companies that wish to manufacture generic medications must show the FDA that their versions are bioequivalent to the brand medications. Bioequivalent means equally potent, pure, stable, processed, and excreted.[112] Nearly half of all prescription medications purchased in the U.S. are generic.[113]

However, generics aren't always perfect substitutes for the branded versions. A 2004 study revealed that patients with epilepsy who switched from a branded anti-seizure medication to the generic equivalent had more seizures requiring hospitalization and emergency room or office visits. Although the FDA found the two versions to be equivalent when the generic version was approved in 1998, real world conditions, like whether the medication was taken with food, may have caused differences in effectiveness.[114]

A case like this is the exception. In general, generics are just as effective as their branded counterparts. One should not forget that many of the current generic medications started out as very popular branded medications. Some, like omeprazole (Prilosec) and loratadine (Claritin) are now even available over the counter.

Only after a branded medication's patent expires can another company produce a generic version. Although patent protection lasts seventeen years, pharmaceutical companies usually have less time than that to market their product exclusively, because patents are filed when a new compound is discovered. That usually occurs years before a drug is refined, tested, and ready for medicinal use. Consequently, the amount of time a manufacturer has to promote its product is shortened.

Once a patent on a medication has expired, companies find other ways to extend the usefulness of their product. They modify the medication slightly to get a new patent. They can also combine it with another medication to form a brand new combination medication.

The FDA maintains a list of medications about to go generic. Its list of approvals and more about generic drugs is at the Office of Generic Drugs at www.fda.gov/cder/ogd. For an unbiased view of prescription medications, review the *Consumer Reports* website at www.crbestbuydrugs.org. Users can download a two-page summary report that lists various medications by class, dosage, and price. The site also offers more comprehensive, detailed reports that are easy to read. Best of all, the website identifies proven therapies, and the information is free. It provides valuable information on medication costs and effectiveness.

Your goal should be to take medication only when necessary and to take medications that are effective, safe, and affordable. There are certain situations, however, when only a branded, and thus more expensive, medication will do. Sometimes there are no alternatives, generic or otherwise, to a particular medication. It may be the only one in its drug class or the only one that provides the desired benefit. In other situations (for example, when treating cancer), the newest medication can make the difference between life and death. When no generic equivalent exists or alternatives do not come close to offering effective treatment, a branded medication must be considered.

Consumers who have no prescription drug coverage, are not eligible for Medicare, meet certain income limits, and are legal residents of the U.S. should look into TOGETHER RX ACCESS program (www.togetherrxaccess.com), a program sponsored by pharmaceutical companies that can provide discounts off certain prescription drugs. Since the group does not include all companies, you may want to review or take a look at individual pharmaceutical companies' websites to see if they also have their own patient assistance programs.

Unless you have a frank discussion with your doctor about medications and their costs, you may be paying more for treatments that may not be better than less pricey alternatives.

PARTNERING WITH YOUR DOCTOR: HAVING A FRANK DISCUSSION

As I discussed earlier, the second largest expense for patients is medication. And since pharmaceutical companies spend the vast majority of their marketing dollars to educate doctors about new and more expensive products, unless you have a frank discussion with your doctor about medications and their costs, you may be paying more for treatments that may not be better than less pricey alternatives. Think about asking your doctor the following questions:

➤ Is it necessary that I take medication?

➤ Is it essential that I take this particular brand or product?

➤ Is this medication proven to be effective for my condition?

➤ Are there other less expensive alternatives that are equally effective?

Physicians are aware that people want to have these discussions. One survey noted that 63 percent of patients wanted to discuss out-of-pocket costs, and 79 percent of physicians believed that patients generally wanted to have this discussion. The reality, however, is that just over a third of physicians and only 15 percent of patients ever had this talk. Your silence may be costing you. Speak up!

What you say can influence your doctor's prescribing habits.

Consider taking free samples from your doctor only if the amount given is enough to take care of your problem. If the medication is for a chronic condition, you should avoid getting a sample. Pharmaceutical companies offer samples to promote their new medications. Once patients sample the medication and rely on it to stay healthy, they become dependent on these treatments.

Distributing free samples is a good way to get new customers, but unlike trial samples of soaps, detergents, lotions, and perfumes, medications can cause serious side effects. Medications should always be treated with more respect and skepticism than free lotion samples. Feel comfortable telling your physician that you aren't interested in free samples and want treatment that is proven, not new.

Believe it or not, what you say can influence your doctor's prescribing habits. One study showed that patients who requested either an advertised or non-advertised prescription medication were much more likely to receive that medication than a patient who didn't suggest a particular medication. But when physicians were asked how likely it was that they would prescribe the same medication to a similar patient with the same ailment who had not requested a specific medication, physicians were ambivalent. Forty percent of the time, physicians were not as confident in their choice if a patient asked for a specific medication (advertised or non-advertised) and were even more ambivalent, 50 percent of the time, when the request was for an advertised medication.[115]

The particular brand of medication you receive may also be determined by your insurance plan. Most insurance companies contract with various pharmaceutical companies to get a cheaper rate by promising to buy large volumes of certain medications. These medications will be on the insurance plan's list of preferred medications, also known as the drug formulary. The insurance plan will require your doctor to prescribe medications listed on the formulary.

If your physician feels that the options on the formulary are not adequate to treat your medical problem, he requests in writing that the insurance company pay for an alternative medication not on the list. If the insurance plan feels that the reason for the change is appropriate, it will cover the cost. If it feels that it is not, you, the patient, will be stuck with the cost.

Pharmaceutical representatives understand this process very well. Not only do they educate physicians about which insurance plans list their products, but they also provide pre-printed forms that physicians simply sign to request that non-participating insurers cover a particular medication. Only if the request is denied does the patient ever learn the true costs of prescription medications. Therefore, if you are concerned about your medication costs, initiate the discussion. Unless you bring it up, your doctor probably won't.

MAKING SENSE OF OVER-THE-COUNTER (OTC) MEDICATIONS

Informed consumers know how to interpret over-the-counter medication labels. Informed consumers compare different brands by cost and content, and understand what the active ingredients are. The labeling includes sections on Drug Facts, Uses, Warnings, Directions, Other Information, and Inactive Ingredients. By reading the labels, you may discover that some of your medications at home already treat the same symptoms as another combination medication.

The Drug Facts section has three important parts: the active ingredient, the amount per unit (i.e. tablet, capsule, teaspoon), and the purpose of the medication. The active ingredients are always written as the chemical or generic name. For the allergy medication Claritin, for example, the Drug Facts will list loratadine, the chemical or generic name, as the active ingredient.

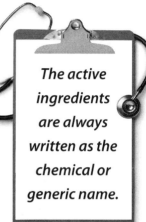

The active ingredients are always written as the chemical or generic name.

Following is a list of potential medications you may encounter. I list the chemical or generic name first and the adult version dosages.

Pain Relievers

Acetaminophen. Many of us know it by its trade name, Tylenol (owned by McNeil Consumer Healthcare). It is a pain reliever and can also reduce fever. It is not an anti-inflammatory. Dosages vary but often will be in 200 mg, 325 mg (regular strength), and 500 mg (extra strength) forms.

Ibuprofen. People commonly interchange the word ibuprofen with its trade names, Motrin and Advil (the former is owned by McNeil Consumer and Specialty and the latter by Wyeth Consumer Healthcare). Ibuprofen comes in 200 mg strength tablets. Ibuprofen can reduce pain and fever, and is also an anti-inflammatory. Dosages in combination medications vary.

Naproxen. Naproxen's trade name is Aleve (owned by Bayer Healthcare). Like ibuprofen, naproxen is a pain reliever and an anti-inflammatory, but chemically it is different from ibuprofen. Over-the-counter, naproxen comes in 200 mg strength tablets.

Caffeine. Caffeine, a stimulant, appetite suppressant, and pain reliever, is used in a variety of medications. It's often found in medications used to treat migraines and headaches.

Decongestants

Pseudoephedrine. Commonly known as Sudafed. As a decongestant, it can open nasal passages and relieve a stuffy nose. Pseudoephedrine has been taken off drug store shelves and placed behind the pharmacy counter as some people were using it to produce methamphetamines. Consumers willing to purchase it must ask a pharmacist for it, are required to sign for it, and are limited to a small number of pills. Because of this restriction, many combination cold and allergy formulations are instead using phenylephrine as their decongestant. The dosage strength varies depending on the formulation. Side effects of either decongestant can include elevated blood pressure, palpitations, and jitteriness.

Antihistamines

Diphenhydramine. Commonly known as Benadryl (owned by Pfizer Inc.). Antihistamines are used to treat allergies, can dry up a runny nose, and decrease symptoms of itchiness. Typical dosages are 25 mg and 50 mg. Side effects can include dry mouth, sleepiness, and problems with urination for men with enlarged prostates.

Chlorpheniramine. Dosages are often 4 mg and 8 mg. Side effects are similar to those of diphenhydramine.

Loratadine. Previously, loratadine was sold as the prescription allergy medication Claritin (owned by Schering-Plough HealthCare Products Inc.). Once it became generic, and because of its safety, it is now sold over the counter. Unlike diphenhydramine and chlorpheniramine, loratadine is less likely to cause sedation.

Cough Medications

Dextromorphan. Dextromorphan is found in many over-the-counter cold or cough medications. The packaging may say "DM."

Guaifenesin. Guaifenesin, the active ingredient in the cough
medication Robitussin (owned by Wyeth Consumer
Healthcare), is a mucolytic. A mucolytic is an ingredient that
loosens phlegm.

With this list of commonly encountered active ingredients, you can
compare products made by the same or different manufacturers. Medications with the same active ingredient and same dosages should give
you the same benefit. Once you have determined that the contents are
the same, pick the one that fits your budget.

Some words of caution: *although over-the-
counter medications are relatively safe, they can still
cause serious medical problems.* Pay particular attention to the Warning and Directions sections of
the Drug Facts label. For example, the warning for
diphenhydramine, in Benadryl, suggests that men
with enlarged prostates who have trouble urinating
should check with their doctor before taking the medication. In some cases, the medication can cause patients
to retain urine, which backs up and produces swelling
in the kidneys, requiring a trip to the doctor's office
where a catheter is placed in the bladder to alleviate the
problem. This particular side effect is in fact common
to many allergy medications with antihistamines.

Don't take too much of any over-the-counter medication. Read and understand the labeling on the package. This can mean the difference between life and death.

Patients who are pregnant or have high blood
pressure, diabetes, glaucoma, and asthma, as well as those who take
prescription medications regularly, should exercise extra caution when
taking over-the-counter medications. If you aren't sure which medications can be taken safely, check with your doctor or pharmacist.

Don't take too much of any over-the-counter medication. Read and
understand the labeling on the package. This can mean the difference
between life and death. For example, the infant version of acetamino-

phen, which comes with a dropper, is much more concentrated than the children's suspension version. If the infant version were given to a child, the resultant dosage would be three times as strong, and could cause serious liver damage or death.

Although over-the-counter medications are fairly safe and don't cause serious side effects, they are not candy and can do real harm when not taken in the proper dosages. Some adults take more than the recommended dosage on the packaging and even exceed the maximum dosage deemed safe by the manufacturer and FDA. *This is dangerous.* If you are not having an adequate response to an over-the-counter medication, don't ignore and disregard the product labeling. Instead, check with your doctor and find out if there is a more effective medication for you.

Note that sometimes you may inadvertently take too much of an over-the-counter medication. This is often possible with the pain reliever acetaminophen, which is included in many cold medications, sleep aids, and allergy treatments, in addition to prescription pain medications. Too much acetaminophen can damage the liver or cause liver failure or even death. Identify which products have acetaminophen and check with your doctor if you are taking too much. For healthy adults, up to 4,000 mg in a twenty-four-hour period is generally safe, while in patients who drink alcohol regularly or have liver problems the number is usually 2,000 mg per day.

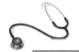 **Real-Life Example**

> Ms. Jones is a twenty-one-year-old woman who suffers from daily headaches, occasional migraine headaches, and periodic hay fever. She uses Excedrin pain reliever, Excedrin tension headache, and Excedrin migraine headache over-the-counter medications. At times she takes

the sleep medications Unisom or Excedrin PM to help her with her insomnia. If her allergies really flare up, she'll try Benadryl.

Reviewing her medications revealed that Ms. Jones was taking the following active ingredients. Below is a list of the active ingredients in Ms. Jones's medications.

Excedrin:

Extra Strength, per tablet: acetaminophen 250 mg, aspirin 250mg, caffeine 65 mg

Tension Headache: acetaminophen 500 mg, caffeine 65 mg

Migraine Headache: acetaminophen 250 mg, aspirin 250mg, caffeine 65 mg

PM: acetaminophen 500 mg, diphenhydramine 38 mg[116]

Unisom Sleep Gel: diphenhydramine 50 mg[117]

Benadryl: diphenhydramine 25 mg[118]

Ms. Jones could eliminate either Excedrin Extra Strength or Excedrin Migraine, as they have identical ingredients, in identical amounts, in each pill. She would only need one product to handle both of her problems. And choosing the drug store/supermarket brand might save her even more money.

The Excedrin PM that she uses to help her sleep contains the pain reliever acetaminophen and the antihistamine diphenhydramine. Although the diphen-hydramine is listed as a nighttime sleep aid, it is the side effect of sedation that is being used to help with sleep. If she has no pain and just wants to get good sleep,

> choosing the Unisom might be better. It has more of the
> sleep aid and no other medications. Finally, her allergy
> medication, Benadryl, has the same active ingredient as
> Unisom and Excedrin PM.

Next time, see for yourself. Examine over-the-counter medications and compare the different allergy, cold, and headache formulations to see what they have in common. See how much you might save by selecting a different brand or a generic brand. Go through your medicine cabinet and see what you already have: search for medicines which are essentially identical, and those that are expired and need to be thrown out. You might be surprised. By the way: expired medications shouldn't be casually thrown away or flushed down the toilet, where their chemicals can enter the water supply and lead to all kinds of environmental problems. Unless the medication insert notes the medication can be safely flushed, it is recommended to remove the medications from the original bottle, mix them with unpalatable substances like coffee grinds or kitty litter, and disposing the contents in a closed bag or an unlabeled can. Many cities have facilities for safe disposal of medications. Check with your pharmacist as well for other options.

Curious what's in other well-known over-the-counter medications? Here are a few more brand names and their common ingredients.

Robitussin

Cough Gels: dextromethorphan 15 mg

Cough and Cold Caplets: dextromethorphan 10 mg, pseudoephedrine 30 mg, guaifenesin 200 mg

DM Cough Syrup: dextromethorphan 10 mg, guaifenesin 100 mg (per teaspoon)

DM Cough Syrup Long Acting: dextromethorphan 15 mg (per teaspoon)[119]

Sudafed

Nasal Decongestant: pseudoephedrine 30 mg

Sinus and Cold: acetaminophen 325 mg, pseudoephedrine 30 mg

Sinus Headache: acetaminophen 500 mg, pseudoephedrine 30 mg

Severe Cold: acetaminophen 500 mg, pseudoephedrine 30 mg, dextromethorphan 15 mg[120]

Tylenol

Regular Strength: acetaminophen 325 mg (per tablet)

Extra Strength: acetaminophen 500 mg

PM: acetaminophen 500 mg, diphenhydramine 25 mg[121]

The FDA, through its Center for Drug Evaluation and Research (CDER), has helpful information about over-the-counter medications, prescription medication, and antibiotic resistance, as well as tips for purchasing medication outside the U.S. and via the Internet. Visit its website at www.fda.gov/cder/audiences. Look for the link labeled Consumer Education: What You Need to Know to Use Medicine Safely.

To learn more about over-the-counter and prescription medications go to www.medlineplus.gov and click on the Drug and Supplements Section. It lists a description of many medications, as well as information about how they work, precautions, safe usage, and side effects. Medications as well as herbal and dietary supplements are included in the database. The website also contains information on a few hundred health topics and has a medical encyclopedia and medical dictionary.

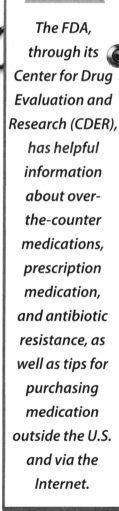

The FDA, through its Center for Drug Evaluation and Research (CDER), has helpful information about over-the-counter medications, prescription medication, and antibiotic resistance, as well as tips for purchasing medication outside the U.S. and via the Internet.

TAKE-HOME POINTS

➤ Pharmaceutical companies spend the vast majority of their marketing on physicians. There are a few places now that prohibit physicians from accepting gifts from representatives in an effort to keep physicians objective.

➤ A small number of branded medications accounts for nearly half the money spent on medications. Sales are rising due to a trend toward higher priced drugs as well as an increased number of medications prescribed.

➤ Nearly half of all prescription medications purchased are generics. Generics must be as potent, pure, stable, processed, and excreted as the branded medication. When available, they can be a good substitute and as effective as a more expensive branded medication.

➤ Talk frankly with your doctor about medication costs and effectiveness. Your physician might not mention it unless you bring it up.

➤ Understanding how to interpret over-the-counter medication labels allows you to compare different brands. This can help you save money, and decreases your chance of taking too much of a medication that can have major side effects.

➤ Learn more about over-the-counter and prescription medications at www.medlineplus.gov. Click on the Drug and Supplements Section.

PART SIX:

Caveat Emptor, Or "Let the Buyer Beware"

> If it sounds too good to be true, it probably is.
>
> "Unless there are credible scientific studies to support these calorie-burning claims, they may be nothing more than voodoo nutrition… Promise of wondrous weight loss must be supported by science, not magic."[122]
>
> — **Connecticut Attorney General Richard Blumenthal announcing investigation of a beverage that claims to provide negative calories.**

When it comes to your health, there are plenty of people willing to offer products and services. Are they worth your hard-earned money or time? Often it's very hard to tell. But once you're fully informed, you can decide what's right for you.

CONCIERGE CARE

When you think of a concierge, you think about a fancy hotel staff person who answers questions, speaks various languages; and books reservations to restaurants, events, and tours, even sold-out attractions — right? The hotel concierge is your insider, someone who possesses intimate knowledge of the city and recommends must-see

Patients in boutique or concierge care pay a retainer ranging anywhere from a few hundred to a few thousand dollars per year.

sites like a true local. You are personally cared for and pampered.

Imagine, then, your physician providing the same attentive service. Indeed, a small and growing number of physicians are offering this concierge care, also known as boutique or retainer medicine. Physicians provide services typically not covered by their traditional health insurance, like annual comprehensive physicals and direct access to their doctors twenty-four hours a day via home phones, cell phones, and pagers. Other benefits include same day appointments with longer physician face time, little to no waiting time in the lobby, and a focus on preventive care. In some practices, the physician will even accompany a patient to specialty doctor appointments and perform house calls. Sound pretty nice? But beware: this kind of service comes at a price. Patients in boutique or concierge care pay a retainer ranging anywhere from a few hundred to a few thousand dollars per year.

The concept of boutique care may have started in 1996, when the Seattle Supersonics former team physician wanted to make available to the general public the same level of medical care and attention provided to professional athletes.[123] MD2, the company he founded, provided a spa-like experience to a select few patients who could afford the $10,000 to $20,000 annual retainer fee (in addition to insurance premiums and costs).[124]

Many physicians are attracted to this new physician-patient relationship as they become more disenchanted with large patient panel sizes, lower reimbursement rates, shorter office visits, increasing overhead, malpractice costs, and paperwork. They want to slow down and spend more time with patients, which is difficult in the current climate of falling insurance reimbursement.[125] In the July 2002 issue of The Journal of Family Practice, one study noted that 27 percent of physicians anticipated a moderate to definite likelihood of leaving their practices within two years. Leland Kaiser, Ph.D., a healthcare futurist, also notes that lack of physician accessibility and availability is also causing consumer discontent and is a driving force toward concierge medicine. He predicts that 30 to 40 percent of all doctor visits in the next decade will be concierge medicine visits.[126]

The high retainer fees these physicians charge frees them financially from health insurance contracts and allow them to care for a much smaller patient panel (typically a third or less than an average physician's panel of two to three thousand patients). Perhaps not surprisingly, these practices attract patients who are upper middle class, middle-aged entrepreneurs, and wealthy seniors.[127]

Supporters of concierge care claim it's a lot like private school education. Parents who wish to supplement their children's education can send them to private school, paying extra for a potentially more personalized education that offers more choices (at a cost). "Like education, luxury primary care is simply a response to a market need [that] serves the interests of both the consumers (patients) and suppliers (physicians)."[128] As long as there are people willing to pay extra for additional personalized care, the more likely the boutique medicine trend will continue.

Concierge care is not just limited to individual physicians. In August 2003, the Boston Globe reported that Tufts University's New England Medical Center, an academic teaching hospital, was providing a concierge practice for $1,800 per year per person.[129] Although boutique medicine was initially confined to Seattle and Florida, it continues to gain followers in about two dozen states, with more than two hundred boutique practices in California. 2004 saw the formation of the American Society of Concierge Physicians.[130,131,132]

Understandably, not everyone is happy about this new trend. While the American Medical Association (AMA) has not found concierge practices to be inconsistent with the goal of healthcare delivery, it bears repeating that a physician's duty is first and foremost to his patients. So, as in the case with physicians who retire or leave a practice, doctors planning on changing to or adopting a new concierge practice need to help their former patients transition to other healthcare providers. If no other physicians in the community are able to care for these patients, the AMA notes that the original physician may be ethically obligated to continue care.

State and federal healthcare agencies, as well as insurance companies, are watching the new developments carefully to ensure that physicians practicing boutique medicine do not require retainers to provide services already covered by a patient's health insurance. In July 2003, the government took action and fined a physician over $50,000 after he charged his patients $600 for services partially covered by Medicare.[133] In 2004, the Health and Human Services Federal Agency reiterated the long-standing policy that physicians are not allowed to charge Medicare patients additional fees for services already covered in the Medicare program. The private health plan Harvard Pilgrim Health Care refused to allow three concierge physicians into its network because it expected that doctors who participated in the network should provide twenty-four-hour access and same-day appointments when appropriate and not charge extra for those services. Many concierge physicians opt to drop all health insurance participation to avoid running afoul of regulators and insurers.

Although concierge patients may feel they are receiving higher quality health care because they have more physician time and attention, there is no scientific evidence at this time to support that assumption. On the contrary, it is possible that as the doctor spends more time caring for fewer patients, his clinical skills may worsen because of decreased volume and exposure to different patients.[134]

If your physician starts to practice concierge medicine, understand that any future contact with your physician may require payment or a retainer prior to you receiving any additional care or service not covered by insurance. Since most concierge physicians are no longer paid by insurance companies, this cost comes directly to you. And if you choose not to continue care, it is your physician's responsibility to help you find another doctor.

Should you take part in a concierge practice? It depends. If you can afford it and you enjoy the personal attention and pampering, concierge medical care might be right for you. Your physician is on a retainer and essentially is on your payroll as a paid consultant. Direct access to your doctor, long comprehensive office visits, and same-day appointments can't be beat.

Or can it? With a bit more time and energy, you can get similar care for less money. Instead of an hour-long consultation with a concierge doctor, you could get the same amount of face time with your regular doctor over a period of three to four separate office visits. The latter would certainly be more inconvenient, however.

The bottom line is that only you can determine how much the extra convenience of concierge care is worth. The lowest retainer for concierge care runs about $600 per person per year. If your current office co-pay costs $20 to $30 per visit, you could see your regular doctor twenty to thirty times for the same amount of money. And if you maximize your office visit, as I discussed earlier, approaching your doctor with a focused agenda instead of a laundry list, you will have an even better experience. Also be aware that more and more physicians are working on open-access scheduling. This system focuses on providing patients with same-day appointments, which has improved satisfaction among patients and physicians.[135] With more physicians adopting this mindset, the same-day access benefit touted by concierge medicine may be less of a deciding factor.

Will concierge medicine be successful? Time will tell.

BODY SCANS

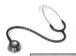 **Real-Life Example**

A couple of years ago, Ms. Smith hobbled in with her cane, angrily waving a sheath of papers with her free hand. She was an otherwise healthy older individual, and I had seen her before for many minor ailments.

"Dr. Liu, I just spent over $1,000 for this body scan!" she said. "The doctors told me that I have a lung mass. They told me it might be cancer and I needed to see you to figure out what it is."

Sure enough, the beautifully typed reports described a small half-inch spot on her upper right lung. Determining the potential causes of a single lung mass was a typical medical student homework assignment. While it could be cancer, there was a long list of other possibilities. Aside from this one spot, the remainder of the CT scan was normal and Ms. Smith felt well. Unfortunately, with the report, we could not simply ignore this mass. So I referred her to a pulmonologist, a lung specialist, for further care.

Two years and four repeat CT scans later, Ms. Smith still hobbled into the office. She wearily plopped herself onto the examination table and sighed about how difficult it was to get older. The pulmonologist had recommended a lung biopsy, but she flatly refused, not wanting to have chest surgery. Instead she opted for careful observation and repeat CT scans. The good news was the lung mass hadn't increased in size or changed in shape.

Aside from being irradiated with four additional CT scans, multiple visits with a specialist, and a lot of worry, Ms. Smith still had a lung mass that was not causing her any problems. Was the body scan worth it?

Over the past few years, many offices and businesses have been promoting the use of body scans. You hear and see their ads on the radio or in the newspaper. For just a few hundred dollars you can buy yourself peace of mind by undergoing a painless, quick imaging test. Scan your internal organs just to make sure you do not have a silent cancer time bomb waiting to explode and end your life prematurely. Look at your heart and your lungs before you have symptoms of chest pain and shortness of breath to make sure those years of smoking and drinking when you were in your twenties did not damage your body. The ads feature testimonials from grateful clients who prolonged their own lives by getting body scans and discovering cancers and other abnormalities that they claim might have been fatal if they hadn't caught them.

Body scans have been called by the Wall Street Journal the biggest craze in preventive medicine since vitamin C.[136] Like Superman's x-ray vision and the medical handheld tri-corders used by the Star Trek medical doctors, these scanners spark the imagination and allow us to look inside our bodies. Patients lie down and are passed thorough a ring of x-ray detectors known as a CT (computed tomography) or CAT (computerized axial tomography) scanner. A computer takes these x-ray images and reassembles them to reproduce a cross-sectional image of the body for a radiologist to interpret. Since the 1970s, this technology has been and continues to be a valuable tool for physicians to diagnose illnesses, plan for treatment, and provide follow-up care. Everyone agrees that CT scanners are very helpful.

The controversy is when to use them. Prior to body scans, patients would only undergo CT scans if their doctors felt it was necessary to clarify a diagnosis or determine a treatment plan. A CT scan was and still is a diagnostic tool and was never intended to be a screening tool. In fact, in April 2002 the FDA reported that it knew of no evidence that whole-body CT scanning was effective in the detection of any disease early enough to prevent a major serious illness or premature death. Additionally, the FDA has never approved CT scanning to be used as a screening procedure.[137]

Proponents of body scans argue that potential cancers and heart disease can be detected years earlier than when using traditional methods of screenings and testing. They argue that unlike current screening tests like flexible sigmoidoscopies, colonoscopies, and mammograms, all of which are either invasive or uncomfortable, body scans do not require patients to disrobe or endure much discomfort. HealthView, one of the first body scan centers in the nation, notes in their advertising that their body scan can uncover asymptomatic and often life-threatening disease generally not detectable by physical exam or standard screening tests. This allows for management of disease at earlier stages, where medical therapy and treatment options are less costly and invasive.[138]

Other advocates say that patients may be more motivated to take better care of themselves if they could see how their lifestyle affected their bodies. A comprehensive body scan takes cross-sectional images of the body starting from the neck and ending at the pelvis. The x-ray pictures are then reviewed by a radiologist, who often discusses the findings with the client and determines which further tests or referrals are needed.

For the most part, body scans are not covered by insurance plans and prices can range from $750 to $1,600. In some instances, insurance plans may cover a portion of the cost if the patient has had a physician referral. You would need to check with your health plan prior to the scan.

For many in the medical community, the risks of body scans far outweigh the benefits. Aside from the fact that body scans expose patients to about 150 times the radiation of a normal chest x-ray,[139] whole body scans are more likely to identify various abnormal findings in a healthy person that will necessitate further work-up. This often requires additional tests and can include invasive procedures. In the majority of cases, these confirmatory tests are normal anyway. So, after an abnormal body scan, an individual may worry needlessly, require additional costly testing, and then ultimately be told that the tests were all normal.

> *Body scans expose patients to about 150 times the radiation of a normal chest x-ray.*

In January 2002 medical expert and doctor Timothy Johnson, preparing for a segment on body scans for ABC's *20/20*, underwent a CT scan that showed a calcified plaque in an artery of his heart. After additional testing, additional radiation, and a cost of $4,000 to his insurance company, the end result was that his heart was fine.[140]

Neither the American College of Radiology, the American College of Cardiology/American Heart Association, the U.S. Preventive Services Task Force, nor the American Cancer Society recommend CT screening.[141,142] In general, doctors are conservative and don't want to do more harm than good. Before recommending body scans, the medical community wants scientific evidence that CT scans actually save lives when used as screening tools. A screening test or procedure is considered valid and effective when it can detect a disease early enough so that treatment changes the outcome and improves the health of an individual.

This is not the first time physicians tried to use a diagnostic test as a screening test. In the 1970s, chest x-rays were being used by the Mayo Clinic on asymptomatic smokers as a way of detecting early lung cancer. They compared this group with another cohort of smokers who received the usual medical care. After following the patients for over twenty years, researchers concluded that although more lung cancers were detected earlier and more surgeries were performed in the group screened with regular chest x-rays, the outcome was the same. Both groups died of lung cancer at the same rate. As a result, routine chest x-rays were no longer recommended as a way of screening for lung cancer. Currently, the National Institutes of Health is studying the use of CT scanning as a method for detecting lung cancer, but the results will not be known for at least seven years.[143]

Although body scans are not as invasive as traditional tests, they may also not be as accurate. One scientific study compared standard colonoscopy with virtual colonoscopy to screen for colon cancer. Virtual colonoscopy, like body scans, uses a CT scanner. A December 2003 report showed the 3D radiological reconstruction by a CT scanner was as sensitive in detection of colon polyps as traditional colonoscopy. Colon polyps (potential precursors to colon cancer) greater than ten millimeters (a little less than half an inch) were detected with the virtual colonoscopy 93 percent of the time. With conventional colonoscopy, they were detected 87 percent of the time.[144] While the virtual colonoscopy was less invasive and less risky, patients with polyps still needed to undergo a conventional colonoscopy to biopsy and remove the growths. The limitation of the study was that it used a novel 3D approach that was only available at the University of Wisconsin.[145]

A report in the Journal of the American Medical Association reported four months later that virtual colonoscopy was not yet accurate enough to replace conventional colonoscopy. The study on which JAMA based its findings involved nine major medical centers; patients all had a virtual colonoscopy before a conventional colonoscopy. It showed that virtual colonoscopy detected ten-millimeter sized polyps only 55 percent of the time while standard colonoscopy detected them 100 percent of the time. The detection rates of the virtual colonoscopy varied among the nine medical centers and did not improve as the study progressed. The authors thus concluded that the virtual colonoscopy is not quite ready for routine use.[146]

Another discussion surrounds the use of electron beam CT (EBCT) to assess the potential risk of heart disease by determining the amount of calcium deposited in a person's coronary artery. A large amount of calcium indicates a large amount of plaque, or a narrowing, of a coronary artery. With that information, the EBCT generates a score that can help predict an individual's risk of having a coronary event within ten years. A high score indicates an increased likelihood of a coronary event like heart attack leading to death, nonfatal heart attack, and cardiac catheterization.

The most recent study on coronary calcium scores suggests that asymptomatic patients in the intermediate risk category, as defined by the National Cholesterol Education Program (NCEP), could consider EBCT as an option to determine their risk further and take appropriate preventive measures.[147] The intermediate risk category includes 40 percent of American adults over age twenty. Supporters feel that using these scores provides patients with another tool to help determine their risk.

However, opponents point out that patients defined as intermediate risk by NCEP guidelines, which does not include a coronary calcium score, will already be started on preventive therapies to decrease their risk of having a coronary event. Interventions like lowering cholesterol and blood pressure, known risk factors for heart disease, would already be in place.

Furthermore, the understanding of the progression of heart disease and heart attacks has been changing. In the past, it was believed that

> *With no evidence-based research that shows these body scans change or improve health outcomes, the boring advice (blood pressure control, use of cholesterol medication, cessation of smoking, and taking aspirin) may be more effective in preventing heart attacks.*

gradual plaque or cholesterol buildup, which is predicted by the coronary calcium score, was the cause of heart attacks. Researchers have discovered, however, that for 75 to 80 percent of heart attack cases, blockage of the coronary artery was not due to gradual cholesterol build up but rather to a piece of plaque present in a relatively normal artery that suddenly broke free and blocked the artery completely.[148]

Based on this new understanding, increasingly popular and aggressive treatments like cardiac stenting and opening narrow clogged arteries may do little or nothing to prevent heart attacks. Individuals could still be at risk for heart disease and heart attacks regardless of their calcium score. A stunning 2007 report showed that in patients with non-emergent symptoms of heart disease, the use of heart stents with maximal medication therapy did no better than medication therapy alone for decreasing the risk of death, heart attack, stroke, or future hospitalization for a repeat heart attack.[149] With no evidence-based research that shows these body scans change or improve health outcomes, the boring advice (blood pressure control, use of cholesterol medication, cessation of smoking, and taking aspirin) may be more effective in preventing heart attacks.[150]

Deciding whether to have a whole body scan is an individual choice. Although there will always be testimonials about how body scans save lives, rarely do we hear about the unnecessary worry and additional testing endured by individuals who had abnormal body scans and later found out they were perfectly healthy.

CT scans are used routinely in patient care. A CT scan may be helpful if someone is suffering from unexplained weight loss, has an abnormal chest x-ray, or is an older patient suffering from a debilitating headache after head trauma. A CT scan may help determine that the person mysteriously losing weight has pancreatic cancer, that an abnormal chest x-ray is the result of a growth, and that the patient with the headache does not in fact have a brain hemorrhage. But even in patients with these symptoms, a normal CT scan is not always the right test. Weight loss can be due to newly developed diabetes or an overactive thyroid; for either disease, the test of choice would be a blood test. A patient complaining of chest pain and shortness of breath during activity should consider having a nuclear medicine scan to check blood flow to the heart.

Even more common than CT body scans are the roaming mobile medical clinics that offer ultrasounds of the aorta (the large artery located in the chest and abdomen), the heart, the carotids (the large neck arteries), and the leg arteries to check the circulation and evaluate for dilation, weakness, and blockage; and of the wrists and heels to evaluate bone strength for signs of osteoporosis (thinning of the bones). While these tests usually cost no more than a couple of hundred dollars, you may wish to hold on to your money.

Here's why. A patient suffering from a weak heart or congestive heart failure can be diagnosed by a physician after a few questions and a physical examination. Should it be necessary, the doctor will order an echocardiogram and the cost will be paid by the insurance company. It's possible the requested ultrasound will provide a more detailed report than that provided by a mobile medical clinic.

Similarly, if you are concerned about osteoporosis, tell your doctor and he will probably order a dual energy x-ray absorptiometry (DEXA) scan to evaluate the bone strength of the low back and hip and look for signs of osteoporosis and fracture. If the osteoporosis is severe enough to cause fractures, the former will cause back pain and the latter will cause profound disability. One in four women who suffers from a hip fracture due to osteoporosis does not survive beyond the first year of the injury. Therefore, while an ultrasound of the heel or wrist is helpful in determining the bone density in those body parts, it is not nearly as important as knowing the bone density of the hip.

Finally, if you are worried about poor circulation in your legs, your doctor can check your leg and foot pulses rather easily in the office. Without leg or calf pain when walking or occurring all the time at rest, it is unlikely there is any significant blockage in the artery to be worried about.

The best way to avoid extra and unnecessary costs, particularly if you wonder whether you have a certain illness or problem, is to ask your doctor. Explain your concerns. If he feels a CT scan is necessary, he will order one. On the other hand, he may order tests that are more appropriate, minimizing your out-of-pocket costs and exposure to unnecessary radiation. One study estimated that the radiation from a full body scan is equal to the radiation exposure experienced by World War II Japanese nuclear bomb survivors at Hiroshima and Nagasaki one and a half miles away from the blast center.[151] Do you want to expose your body to that kind of radiation unless it's absolutely necessary? If you cannot sleep at night and have your mind completely made up about getting a body scan, go ahead. Just understand the potential risks and problems you might uncover, like Ms. Smith did.

> *One study estimated that the radiation from a full body scan is equal to the radiation exposure experienced by World War II Japanese nuclear bomb survivors at Hiroshima and Nagasaki one and a half miles away from the blast center.*

The process of scanning the whole body in a healthy asymptomatic patient reminds me of my Christmas shopping trips. I have no idea what I'm looking for, but I hope to find something. The vast majority of the times I find nothing. The times I do find something, the recipient usually returns it. Unlike my shopping expeditions, if something is found in a body scan, it must be evaluated all the way to the end. So *caveat emptor* — let the buyer beware.

HERBAL AND DIETARY SUPPLEMENTS

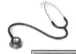 **Real-Life Example**

> Ms. Cook wanted a physical and like many of my patients, she was concerned about staying healthy and preferred not to take any prescription medications, if at all possible. Although she denied taking any medications when asked by my medical assistant, she promptly listed ten to fifteen herbal and dietary supplements when asked directly about using over-the-counter products or vitamins. She was not entirely sure why she was taking them or how they worked but she was certain they were keeping her healthy.
>
> While I applauded her proactive approach toward maintaining/monitoring/taking care of her health, I explained that herbal and dietary supplements, though available over the counter, were not necessarily safe — or the best thing for her. I told her she might be spending a lot of money for unproven therapies.

Dietary supplement producers do not need FDA approval before selling their products.

With the increasing focus on preventive health, rising health care costs, and renewed interest in natural products, it is not surprising that more people are using herbal products to prevent and treat healthcare problems. Herbals and dietary supplements are extremely popular. It's estimated that consumers spend $18 billion annually on the 29,000 products currently available.[152] To put this in perspective, this is nearly the same amount of money spent on video games in 2002 ($10.3 billion) and movie theater tickets ($8.9 billion) combined.[153,154] Their popularity has led to a general perception that natural products are safe and can be taken without side effects. About 59 percent of Americans believe that supplements must be approved by the FDA, the federal agency responsible for overseeing herbal and dietary supplements, and 55 percent believe that health claims for supplements must be backed by solid scientific evidence.[155] But the expectations that these products are as carefully monitored as over-the-counter and prescription medications are deeply misguided.

Most people don't know that the FDA has limited power when it comes to regulation of these herbals or dietary supplements. In 1994, the Dietary Supplement Health Education Act (DSHEA) created regulations regarding the safety and labeling of dietary supplements. The law indicated how ingredients in the product must be labeled and whether or not manufacturers needed to notify the FDA about bringing a "new dietary ingredient" to market. Herbal or dietary supplements marketed prior to October 15, 1994 were not considered new and did not require FDA notification.

As the law currently stands, manufacturers of these products are solely responsible for determining that the dietary supplements they produce and distribute are safe and that claims about their effectiveness are supported by adequate evidence. Manufacturers are not required to register their products (or themselves) with the FDA prior to producing or selling these products. The FDA does not set limits for serving size or the total amount of a particular nutrient in the final product. Unlike manufacturers of prescription drugs, who must prove that the drugs are safe and effective for their intended use, and who must forward to the FDA reports about injuries or illnesses possibly related to their drugs, dietary supplement producers do not need FDA approval before selling their products. This is why all dietary supplements have the disclaimer that these products have not been "evaluated by the FDA for treatment, prevention, or cure" for a specific disease or condition. The FDA has no authority to require any studies of safety or effectiveness for dietary supplements. The burden of proof lies with the FDA to show that a dietary product is "unsafe" before it can restrict use or recall the product from the market.[156]

The current FDA policy regarding dietary nutritional supplements is as follows:

> *FDA regulates dietary supplements under a different set of regulations than those covering "conventional" foods and drug products (prescription and over the counter).* Under the Dietary Supplement Health and Education Act of 1994 (DSHEA), the dietary supplement manufacturer is responsible for ensuring that a dietary supplement is safe before it is marketed. FDA is responsible for taking action against any unsafe dietary supplement product after it reaches the market. Generally, manufacturers do not need to register their products with FDA nor get FDA approval before producing or selling dietary supplements. *Manufacturers*

> *must make sure that product label information is truthful and not misleading.*
>
> FDA's post-marketing responsibilities include monitoring safety, e.g. voluntary dietary supplement adverse event reporting, and product information, such as labeling, claims, package inserts, and accompanying literature. The Federal Trade Commission regulates dietary supplement advertising.[157]

These guidelines aren't particularly reassuring. Without clear regulations, and because there is such a wide variety/range of mixtures of herbal and dietary supplements, there can be large variability in quality of products, both within and among manufacturers. While herbal products labeled with "U.S. Pharmacopoeia" or "National Formulary" comply with DSHEA standards for product quality as defined by the U.S. Pharmacopeial Convention, this is strictly voluntary, which means there may be many adulterated products on the market.[158]

The lack of stringent standards for herbal and dietary supplements and the limited power of the FDA has put the public at risk. Take the example of a Baltimore Orioles rookie baseball player, who died suddenly of heatstroke during spring training in February 2003. His death was linked to use of ephedra.[159] The problems with ephedra were certainly not new or unfamiliar to the FDA. In June 1997, the FDA first proposed that supplements containing ephedra be labeled hazardous and not to be taken for more than seven days. It also suggested restricting the amount of ephedra and combining ephedra with other stimulants in these supplements.[160] While this rule was modified in 2000, it was not until December 2003 that the FDA issued a consumer alert warning the public about the dangers of this product, and not until April 2004 did the FDA finally prohibit the sale of any dietary supplements containing ephedra.[161] By the time of the player's death, the FDA already had reports of 155 deaths and 16,000 complaints related to ephedra.

In November 2004, the FDA warned consumers purchasing the natural impotence product, Actra-Rx, not to take it because it contained prescription strength levels of Viagra.[162] This is particularly troubling since patients taking nitroglycerin or nitrates can have dangerously low blood pressure or heart attacks when taking Viagra. Presumably, those patients, who were not candidates for Viagra because of their heart condition and use of nitroglycerin and nitrates, may have unwittingly harmed themselves more by seeking alternative, nonprescription medications.

While the public may be uncertain about what they're purchasing, they might not be able to rely on their doctors to tell them. The truth is that medical doctors (MDs and DOs) are not adequately prepared to answer questions about safety and usage of these products. One study of family physicians showed that although 87 percent of surveyed physicians had been asked about herbal and dietary supplements, less than half actually could identify side effects of three of the top five herbs most frequently asked about and less than a third of physicians had received any education on these products. Patients disclosed that 41 percent of the time, their source of supplements came primarily from friends and family.[163]

When you consider that there are prescription medication equivalents that have undergone tremendous scrutiny and shown to be effective in clinical trials, why would you want to take a chance with unproven, expensive, and potentially harmful herbal and dietary supplements? A May 2004 Consumer Reports article identified twelve truly harmful herbs that were easily purchased at a store or on the Internet. Five of the supplements have been banned by Canada, Europe, and Asia. One example is aristolochic acid, a product of the Aritsolochia vine, a very powerful toxin that results in kidney failure.[164] Although in 2001, FDA banned further imports of this product, in 2004, products containing the substance were still available for purchase in the United States. Some consumers, after ingesting it, required subsequent kidney transplants and now take multiple prescription medications daily for life.

Not all dietary supplements or herbal medications are bad. A common dietary supplement, lactase, helps patients with lactose intolerance (an inability to digest milk products, causing abdominal bloating and diarrhea). Lactase is found over the counter and is also used to produce lactose-free milk products found in grocery stores. Other helpful therapies include Lactobacillus, the "good" bacteria common in the colon, which when taken regularly can help prevent colon infection caused by "bad" bacteria like *C. difficile*. Glucosamine, a common joint supplement, may help improve arthritis pain.

As researchers continue to investigate different herbal and nutritional supplements, don't be surprised if something that was once touted as helpful later becomes labeled as worthless. The important thing to realize is that until the FDA overhauls its oversight of these products, or until adequate testing of herbal and dietary supplements is performed, you cannot take them with the same level of comfort or safety that you can with prescription and over-the-counter medications.

Until recently, there was no central resource that rated herbal treatments' efficacy. Herbal and dietary products cannot claim to "diagnose, treat, cure, or prevent any disease," because to do so would imply that these products were drugs and consequently would need to comply with more stringent regulations. However, a team at Massachusetts General Hospital is reviewing the existing research studies and determining the validity of the studies. Their findings can be found at www.naturalstandard.com.[103] They hope to provide doctors with useful information about these ingredients, backed by scientific research. Another useful reference is at www.consumerreportsmedicalguide.org.

If you truly want to take an herbal or dietary supplement, enroll in a research study where you are carefully monitored. Read up on the latest research. Purchase products from a reputable manufacturer by checking out the label. Consider taking products that only have one ingredient rather than those with a combination of different substances. Or spend your hard-earned money and precious time on proven therapies, like quitting smoking, exercising, and maintaining a healthy weight.

If an herbal or dietary supplement sounds too good to be true, it probably is.

The bottom line is that if an herbal or dietary supplement sounds too good to be true, it probably is.

Following is a list of some frequently used herbal and dietary supplements, the illnesses they are indicated for, and existing research that proves or disproves their efficacy.

Name	Indications	Research
Echinacea	To prevent and treat colds.	A 2000 study showed that the product had "no significant effect" on the severity or the frequency of developing a cold.[166]
Glucosamine	To decrease and treat arthritis.	In randomized placebo controlled trials, one out of five patients had improved joint mobility and slowed joint space narrowing (more narrowed joint space indicates a more arthritic joint). Side effects were comparable to placebo.[167] A double blind study suggested that combined with chondroitin, glucosamine may be more effective than the placebo in patients with moderate to severe knee pain.[168]
Saw Palmetto	Helps improve urinary flow in men with enlarged prostates.	Clinical trials suggest Saw Palmetto does improve these symptoms.
Kava	To relieve anxiety and stress.	Banned by Canada, Singapore and Germany, as many kava products were linked to liver damage. FDA issued a warning describing the problem. While trials suggest superiority to placebo, caveats remain.
Garlic	To lower cholesterol.	An NIH study in 2001 found that garlic could cause harmful side effects for patients undergoing HIV treatment.

Name	Indications	Research
Vitamin C	An antioxidant.	No research shows Vitamin C can prevent cancer or cardiovascular disease. Observational studies have shown no significant association with risk of breast, prostate, colon, or lung cancer.[169]
Vitamin E	To prevent heart disease.	Studies show no significant benefit in preventing cardiovascular disease. Six of seven trials in patients with cardiovascular disease showed that usage of vitamin E did not significantly reduce cardiac events. A 2004 study noted that patients taking 200 units or more daily had an increased risk of death.[170] A study of nearly 4,000 patients 55 and older over a period of 7 years showed no difference with taking 400 units and placebo. There was an increased likelihood of developing heart failure with vitamin E.[171]
St. John's Wort	For mild depression symptoms.	A 2002 National Institutes of Health (NIH) study showed that the supplement was no more effective than placebo.[172]
Ginkgo	To improve memory.	Was studied and showed no demonstrable benefit in memory in a JAMA study. Other studies suggest superiority to placebo with caveats. When combined with aspirin or warfarin (Coumadin), results in bleeding. Ginkgo by itself has been associated with bleeding.

TAKE-HOME POINTS

There are many exciting new trends in health care and all of us should be aware of them as they will undoubtedly play a role in the future.

✓ *Concierge care may change the way you receive care from your primary care physician.* In this type of practice, your doctor is on an annual retainer ranging in the hundreds to thousands of dollars. The advantage is you get direct access to him twenty-four hours a day, as well as same-day office appointments. There is no evidence that the quality of care is better or worse than in traditional practices.

✓ *Body scans are becoming more commonplace, but there is no research that shows that they save lives.* More often than not, body scans on asymptomatic patients reveal more abnormal findings that require a full medical work up before they are deemed benign. Occasionally they reveal true deadly pathologies. Patients who choose to have body scans do so at their own risk.

✓ *Herbal and dietary supplements,* despite what a majority of Americans think, are not as carefully regulated by the FDA as over-the-counter and prescription medications are. With so many effective medications on the market, patients need to be aware that taking these supplements not only may be ineffective, but also could be expensive and detrimental to their health. Consider not purchasing or ingesting any product with the disclaimer "this product has not been evaluated by the FDA for treatment, prevention, or cure" for a specific disease or condition.

PART SEVEN:

Twenty-First Century Medical Care

According to some economists, by 2016 the amount spent on health care would account for one out of every five dollars spent in the United States, double that from a decade earlier.

Necessity is the mother of all invention.

LOOKING FORWARD: TRENDS REDEFINING HEALTH CARE

Although most of medical school was devoted to teaching students how to be doctors, for me, one lecture stands out. It was about the fundamental challenge of providing health care. To provide health care, one needs to balance three interrelated factors: access, cost, and quality. The unfortunate truth is that only two of the three can be optimized. The third factor is often adversely affected.

If a nation decided that it wanted to provide unrestricted access to all as well as high quality care, it would be at a high cost. If instead it wanted to provide low cost health care and excellent quality, then access would need to be limited, as it would be too expensive. Another possibility would be to provide low-cost health care and improved access, but only by compromising health care quality. The worst scenario would be to provide limited access and low quality at a high cost. This, currently describes our healthcare system. Compared to other industrialized nations, our country has millions of uninsured, one of the highest costs per capita, and worse outcomes.

Despite the truth that only two of the three factors can be done well, it has not stopped physicians and healthcare specialists from trying to find an answer to this seemingly unsolvable question. Some of the innovations that have developed over the past few years try to address this problem. The following trends are more commonplace and rapidly becoming the standard of care. You may experience these in the future.

HOSPITALISTS

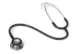 **Real-Life Example**

As I entered the exam room, Mr. Roberts's face lit up. An overweight elderly veteran, he sat on the chair adjacent to the exam table. Mr. Roberts, like many of his generation, smoked and drank years before the medical community knew how detrimental these timeless traditions were to good health. His speech was chronically labored and brief due to emphysema, his legs were always swollen from congestive heart failure, and his hands and feet tingled from nerve damage caused by years of diabetes. Unlike his previous visits, this time his daughter and son accompanied him. Mr. Roberts had been discharged from the hospital about one week prior and was seeing me for follow up.

> Although he was feeling much better, his daughter was concerned that I was not personally caring for her father during his hospitalization. She, like many patients and families, was unfamiliar with hospitalists. She worried that the doctors did not have adequate knowledge about her father or his medical problems and wondered if the hospitalist communicated enough information to ensure a smooth transition from the hospital to home and to his regular doctor.

While a relatively new concept in the United States, the use of hospitalists is common in Canada and Great Britain.[173] Hospitalists are becoming more prevalent due to a combination of medical advances and the demand for efficient and proper care for hospitalized patients. As patients live longer and consequently develop more chronic illnesses, their medical care is more complicated. With continual changes and refinements in medical treatments, it is difficult for primary care physicians to stay current on the latest information to provide their patients the best care both in and out of the hospital. In addition, physicians are pressured by insurers to contain costs and provide efficient care during hospitalization. The traditional model of the primary care physician caring for hospitalized patients before, during, and after office hours does not fulfill these goals.

Hospitalists are much like primary care physicians who efficiently manage and coordinate care for office patients, obtain appropriate specialty referrals, and strive

Hospitalists are much like primary care physicians who efficiently manage and coordinate care for office patients, obtain appropriate specialty referrals, and strive for good health outcomes, except that their office is the hospital.

for good health outcomes, except that their office is the hospital. While some people feel the creation of hospital-based care was primarily driven by managed care to drive down costs, it actually started in 1994 at the Park Nicollet Clinic. Physicians unhappy about the uncertainty of night call and the challenges of working the next day developed what is widely regarded as the first large hospitalist program in the United States.[174]

Proponents argue that hospitalists, by virtue of working in the hospital full time, can coordinate care more quickly and efficiently, decrease hospital costs and lengths of stay, and improve patient care, clinical outcomes, and patient satisfaction. With modern hospital care becoming more demanding, it is also believed that developing hospitalists will provide future generations of physicians with good role models for excellent inpatient care.

There are currently about 8,000 hospitalists in the United States, with projected growth to 20,000 — roughly the same number of cardiologists in the United States.[175] The vast majority are trained in internal medicine and the remainder in family medicine, pediatrics, pulmonary and critical care specialties, or infectious disease. Special post-graduate training programs and fellowships have been established to further advance their medical knowledge and technical skills. In the state of Massachusetts, hospitalist programs manage over 40 percent of medical inpatients. With the present demand for hospitalists growing, there's a good chance that you may be cared for by a hospitalist physician in the future.

The hospital medicine trend, however, does have its critics. The biggest concern is that there might be a disruption in the continuity of care from the office to the hospital. In the past, it was believed that a primary care physician, who was familiar with a patient's medical and personal history, would be best equipped to treat the patient during hospitalization. Instead, with hospital medicine, the patient's care is completely provided by a hospital-based physician, often a complete stranger who's unfamiliar with the patient's medical and personal history. Many predicted that this "handing-off" of patient responsibility would result in worsening outcomes and increasing patient dissatisfaction, particularly if the primary care physician and hospitalist did not communicate.

Research studies so far do not support these concerns. The use of hospitalists has actually led to cost savings, lower rates of repeat hospitalization, shorter hospital stays, decreased hospital and short-term deaths, and improved patient and physician satisfaction and trainee education. While there is no evidence that hospitalists improve the quality of patient care, there is also no proof that patient health care suffers. As the field of hospital medicine develops and matures, research is still ongoing to determine if these benefits will continue.

The bottom line is if you suffer from a chronic illness that makes it likely that you will be hospitalized, find out if your primary care doctor takes care of you in the hospital or partners with a hospitalist. The only time you would ever encounter a hospitalist is if you are ever hospitalized. Your routine office care would still be addressed by your primary care doctor.

Find out the hospitalist's training background by asking your primary care doctor which hospitalist he works with. Does the hospitalist specialize in infectious disease or pulmonary medicine, or is he a generalist in internal or family medicine? Is he a member of the Society of Hospital Medicine (SHM), a professional organization? (Currently, hospital medicine is not recognized as a medical specialty by the American Board of Medical Specialties.) Wise patients know that being cared for by a hospitalist physician has no effect on quality of care, but since the length of stay is shorter, out-of-pocket costs and co-payments may be less expensive.

If you are hospitalized, you want the hospitalist to know you and your medical history quickly and accurately. Be sure to give him the name and office telephone number of your primary care physician so that he can call him to find out more about your past history. Also, be sure to call your primary care doctor to let him know that you have been hospitalized, where you are staying, and the name of the hospitalist. If you have a typed summary of your personal medical history with you as described earlier, this would be a perfect time to use it.

When you are released from the hospital, a discharge summary, a report of the treatments and interventions provided to you in the hospital, is dictated and a copy sent to your primary doctor. If you are asked to follow up with your regular doctor, call his office a day or two before the scheduled appointment to see if his office received the discharge summary. Having the discharge summary can be helpful for your regular doctor to determine why you were in the hospital, what happened while you were there, and what further treatments or tests are necessary to continue to keep you healthy. Often, the hospitalist may have suggestions and recommendations for additional testing or treatments that might be important for future care, but were not needed during the hospitalization.

At the end of our office visit, Mr. Roberts's daughter was relieved to learn that the hospitalist had contacted me about her father's hospitalization and sent me a discharge summary well before Mr. Roberts's office visit with me. I had reviewed the report before entering the room. According to the discharge summary and the examination in the office, Mr. Roberts was much improved.   I ordered a repeat chest x-ray, since the x-ray taken in the hospital showed pneumonia. I reminded him to finish all of the antibiotics. As he slowly pulled himself up with the cane, huffing and puffing, Mr. Roberts smiled and said, "See you next time, Doc!" His daughter and son were glad to see that their father was well taken care of.

GROUP VISITS

Individuals with chronic illnesses like diabetes, congestive heart failure, or emphysema, as well as others who use the healthcare system more than twice a month, may have the opportunity to spend an hour and a half to two hours weekly, biweekly, or monthly with their doctor. They will meet, receive support, and learn from other patients with similar problems. This will be accomplished with the next big thing in health care: the group visit.

Unlike the traditional one-on-one appointment with the doctor, in a group visit patients get together in a group setting and meet with their doctor and a support person. Over the next couple of hours patients have time to ask questions, discover new ideas, receive support from their peers, and understand how to empower themselves. If required, during the visit, the patient can meet privately with the physician. Typically, topics of discussion include common problems related to a particular illness or challenges confronting the participants.

Group visits addressed the problem of increasing panel size, longer wait times, and decreased physician availability, an ever-worsening problem in the United States.

The concept of a group visit is not entirely new. First developed in 1990, the group visit began as an innovative solution to help manage patients who utilized the medical system at high levels. Later, the program was modified to focus on people with chronic diseases. In 1996, another entirely different model developed, which focused less on caring for patients who shared common demographics or ailments and more on an entire physician's patient panel. Group visits addressed the problem of increasing panel size, longer wait times, and decreased physician availability, an ever-worsening problem in the United States.[176]

The initial group visit model, known as the Cooperative Health Care Clinic (CHCC), comes in two types: the CHCC model that focuses on patients who access the healthcare system frequently; and the specialty CHCC model that groups together patients with the same illness. The first type of visit typically enrolls seniors who contact the healthcare system more than two times per month or who use the system frequently. This group of twenty to twenty-five patients meets monthly. Typically a session lasts about two and a half hours, with ninety minutes devoted to group interaction and an hour to patients who wish to see their physician privately.[177] Half of the ninety-minute session is dedicated to various topics, including advance directives, effective use of emergency services, long-term care, and other relevant topics. The remainder of the time is spent on group socialization, bonding, and a question and answer session.

The second type of visit, the specialty CHCC, while similar to CHCC, focuses not on how patients utilize the healthcare system but on certain patient characteristics, like common chronic illnesses. Successful pilot programs for this type of group care have included groups devoted to fibromyalgia, emphysema, irritable bowel syndrome, and congestive heart failure.[178] The goal again is to provide information more efficiently, share knowledge from peers, and improve access to physicians.

Another group visit is the Drop-In Group Medical Appointment (DIGMA). It's a little different than the other two examples. Patients are invited to follow up in the DIGMA after an office visit or when patients are overdue or are on a waiting list for a return appointment. DIGMAs can be thought of as an extended office appointment with a holistic approach. Patients see not only their own physician, but also a behavioral health provider who partners with the doctor.[179] The behavioral health provider is often a psychologist, social worker, marriage and family therapist, nurse, or health educator. DIGMAs, unlike CHCCs are usually weekly or biweekly and last anywhere from one to two hours. Roughly ten to sixteen patients attend with their support people, bringing the total size attending the group to between twelve and twenty-two.

DIGMAs are office visits: the physician is actively taking care of patients by ordering relevant laboratory tests, refilling or changing medications, ensuring that routine maintenance examinations are up to date, and sometimes performing examinations. This improves a physician's office availability because patients who are chronically ill but stable, or those we call the "worried well," are able to see their physicians without using an increasingly scarce resource, the office appointment.[180]

Participation in DIGMAs, like CHCCs, is completely voluntary. These group visits are not designed to replace office visits, but rather to supplement them since traditional office visits may no longer be economically feasible or don't allow the time to address psychosocial or other secondary issues. Office visits are still, however, the appointment of choice for initial patient evaluations, one-time consultations, visits requiring procedures, medical emergencies, acute illnesses, or for patients who refuse group appointments.

There is evidence that group visits work, and that patients and physicians are satisfied with them. Physicians used to repeating the same educational information over and over again in an office visit can have an equal impact by presenting the same information once to a group and still have time left over for additional questions. The interactive nature of the group visit also breaks up the monotony of the office practice. Patients report that the warm, supportive environment of a group visit is "stronger than family" and like "Dr. Welby care".[181] As patients listen to, learn from, and observe their peers, they become more empowered themselves, feel less isolated, and begin to confide in others who truly know what it means to be in their situation.

Research has shown that there are real measurable health advantages to this model as well. One study showed that over a two-year period, among a group of 321 chronically ill older patients, group visit patients had fewer emergency room visits, subspecialist visits, and repeat hospitalizations, as well as greater overall satisfaction with care when compared to a control group.[182] Another study noted that participants in the diabetic group visits had a 32 percent reduction in total cholesterol/HDL ratios, a 30 percent reduction in HgbA1c (a measure that indicates the average blood sugar over a three month period), and a 7 percent reduction in health care expenses. The authors of the study noted that although patients improved their dietary compliance, they sensed that patients seemed more empowered by spending more time with their doctors and getting answers to questions they may never have asked individually, but were willing to ask in a group setting.[183]

 Real-Life Example

> Many of my diabetic patients have shared similar experiences in our diabetic group visits. Those who are having difficulty managing their blood sugar listen and ask questions of those patients who are doing very well. They are encouraged when they meet peers facing similar problems and challenges but who are doing well. Seeing others who suffer from complications like amputations and visual impairment makes the illness much more personal and real than any warnings a physician could offer.
>
> I have a health educator lead my group visit. He changes topics every few months so that participants are always offered new information. I'm also present during the entire visit to answer individual questions, make sure routine laboratory tests are done, and medications are prescribed or refilled.

As patients continue to live longer with chronic illnesses and their demand and utilization for health care increases, patients and physicians can expect to see more of each other in group visits.

EVIDENCE-BASED MEDICINE

In the movie "Jerry McGuire," Cuba Gooding Jr. tells Tom Cruise: "Show me the money!" In many ways, physicians are equally demanding, but instead of money, they want scientific evidence and proof that treatments and proposed interventions work. The phase "evidence-based medicine" was coined by a group of clinicians and epidemiologists in the 1990s to describe the trend of taking results from academia and research studies and applying them to real-world patients and patient care.[184] Prior to that, treatments were often based on anecdotal evidence and tradition.

Take the example of hormone replacement therapy (HRT) for women in menopause. A 2001 review article noted that in observational studies, i.e., a retrospective review of statistics, women who took estrogen had a 35 to 50 percent lower risk of heart disease than women who did not take estrogen. The authors also concluded that while there was an association, there was no proof that taking estrogen decreased the risk as there were no randomized trials, i.e., with a group of patients followed prospectively, that confirmed these observational findings.[185] Nevertheless, for years physicians and patients thought that taking hormone replacement medication could protect menopausal women from heart disease.

Finally, prospective trials were started to see whether hormone replacement therapy was actually beneficial in preventing heart disease. The news was surprising. HRT was shown to increase the risk of heart attacks and other cardiac events. Researchers expected an additional six to eleven cases per year of heart disease for every 10,000 women on HRT.[186] These studies definitively showed that taking HRT did not in fact prevent or protect women from heart disease as previously thought. The findings had tremendous implications for the millions of women on HRT. If women continued to take HRT, then as a nation potentially thousands of extra heart attacks would occur. Understandably, patients, health officials, and the media were concerned about getting the new message out.

Evidence-based medicine is not perfect. While research may show a benefit when a group of patients is studied, the actual outcome for an individual patient depends on a multitude of factors.

Although the evidence is compelling, it applies to a large population. Interpreting information for an individual is not always as easy. Based on the news reports, many of my patients wanted to get off HRT immediately. While I certainly agreed with them, I also pointed out an important fact. The research showed an increase of six to eleven cases per year for every 10,000 women on HRT. That would mean that if I cloned my patient 10,000 times, six to eleven more cases of heart disease might be found among her clones. Therefore, the risk to my individual patient was in fact very, very small. Indeed, the research suggested that women should not take HRT with the goal of preventing heart disease, and it also showed that the risk to an individual was very, very small.

Evidence-based medicine is not perfect. While research may show a benefit when a group of patients is studied, the actual outcome for an individual patient depends on a multitude of factors, including whether an individual's characteristics match those of the studied population (for example, in many research studies most of the participants are white men. Results might not necessarily apply to men of other ethnic backgrounds, or to women), and a little luck.

Let's pretend that you planned a research study to determine the likelihood of rolling a six on a six sided die. You decide to roll a million dice simultaneously and count the number of dice that come up displaying a six. Not surprisingly, your research would conclude that your chance would be one in six.

As you proudly discuss your findings with your friend, he wishes to challenge you on your results. He takes one of your dice and rolls it three consecutive times. To your amazement, each time he rolls it, it turns up with a six. For him, the probability of getting a six was 100 percent. Does that mean your research is wrong or faulty? Absolutely not. Had he continued to roll the die, over time his chance of rolling a six would be one in six. It just so happened that during the time you observed him, he was lucky.

Take another example. I think we can all agree that driving on the highway at one hundred miles an hour is more dangerous than driving at fifty-five miles per hour. Despite this increased risk, it is entirely possible that you could drive everyday at that higher rate of speed and never get into an accident. You can imagine what would happen if everyone drove that fast: there would be an increase in the number of accidents and deaths in the community. But your personal experience might be very different than the experience of the entire population.

Wise patients understand that there is this inherent mismatch between an individual's experience and that of the general population. While studies can show that certain outcomes, interventions, or procedures benefit a group of people, an individual person may not have the same outcome. These studies aren't perfect. On the other hand, basing treatments on evidence is probably better than relying on tradition or what *seems* to make sense.

But even with proven therapies, applying evidence-based medicine does not guarantee positive outcomes. It can only maximize it. I remember meeting Mr. Wellington, a middle-aged man who was undergoing treatment for metastatic colon cancer, the third most lethal cancer in the United States. The research showed that patients can decrease their risk of dying from colon cancer if they undergo sigmoidoscopy screenings, as recommended by the American Cancer Society.

Much to the surprise of Mr. Wellington, his family, and his friends, he focused on staying proactive and keeping healthy. He did not smoke, did not drink, and dutifully did all of the screening tests recommended by his doctor. Nevertheless, he developed an aggressive form of colon cancer that had already spread to his liver. His prognosis was very grim, and he died shortly after my first visit with him. The research only discusses decreasing risk and maximizing benefit. It does not guarantee optimal results.

Informed patients want their doctors to practice medicine based on and backed by evidence and verified by rigorous research rather than on myths or traditions. They realize, however, that these research studies examine large patient populations, and therefore the results might not apply to an individual patient. Only *you* can decide what's best for *you*. If you have doubts about what to do, err on the side of caution and discuss your concerns with your doctor.

TAKE-HOME POINTS

There are many exciting new trends in health care to be aware of. They will undoubtedly play a role in the future.

✓ The use of physicians called **hospitalists** is one of the latest trends in health care. These are dedicated physicians whose office is the hospital, and they care for hospitalized patients. There is some evidence that they provide the same level of care at lower costs and with shorter hospital stays.

✓ **Group visits** are becoming more common as physicians have increasing demands to see more patients and improve access. In the future you may be invited to a group visit composed of peers with a similar illness.

✓ **Evidence-based medicine** is an important concept that was developed in the early 1990s. It refers to applying the results of research into real world day-to-day practice. Patients need to know that although it is important their physicians practice evidence-based medicine, an individual patient can still have an adverse outcome, because evidence focuses on a large population of patients. Clearly, having medical treatments and interventions based on research is far better than having treatments grounded in tradition and anecdotal evidence.

PART EIGHT:

Take Control:
Excellent Health Pays

"In a 10-year study by RAND Corporation ... 25- to 54-year-olds who reported being in "excellent" health at the beginning of the decade saw their median net worth nearly double by the end of the study, to $128,000, while for those with poor health, wealth actually shrunk." [187] — **Smart Money**

SELF-SERVE HEALTH CARE

Health care delivery in America is fundamentally changing. Health care costs are rising much faster than inflation. Employers are unable to stay competitive by absorbing these costs and instead are passing them directly to their employees by reducing health insurance benefits and coverage. Individuals are forced to pay more and given more responsibility about when to get medical care and how to spend their money wisely.

The shifting of responsibility from employer to employee is similar to the trend which has affected retirement plans. The traditional pension plans companies provided their workers started to become too expensive. Thus, over the past few years companies have curtailed and stopped giving out these plans. Instead, workers are asked to contribute more of their own money to retirement and to choose how to invest it.

With health care, not making the right choices today can make the difference between okay health and great health.

Research has shown that large numbers of people are worse off in the new retirement plans. Many do not understand the system, are not saving enough money, or are not investing their money wisely. Their retirement nest eggs are much smaller than they would have been had the pension plans still continued. For some, overcoming their mistakes requires them to delay retirement and work longer.

With health care, not making the right choices today can make the difference between okay health and great health. Unlike retirement planning, one cannot simply get good health by working longer. If there is a lesson to be learned from the change in retirement planning it's that people are not prepared for the change and are worse off than in the previous system. It's reasonable to assume that the same problem will occur with the health-care system. More people will be worse off than in the current system.

Avoid becoming an individual who leaves his health to chance. Protect yourself. Give yourself every edge to stay healthy. Without major reform of the entire healthcare system, the trend of increasing personal responsibility will not change. Take charge now.

Insurance

The most important financial asset you own is your ability to earn money, which ultimately depends on your health. Therefore it is absolutely critical to have some health insurance. Although many of us are tempted not to purchase insurance because of skyrocketing costs, should something happen to you, you may find yourself in financial ruin.

Better than having no insurance would be the purchase of catastrophic health insurance. Catastrophic insurance would help protect you from going bankrupt should you require expensive health care. It is relatively inexpensive as it does not provide coverage for basic healthcare problems.

If you can afford more, then consider the insurance plans with deductibles. Like your auto insurance, you pay full price until you reach the deductible. Once that happens, the insurance company shares the burden of cost. While not as good as the next plan, it is better than catastrophic health insurance as you will have some coverage for less serious medical problems. The newer deductible plans favor individuals who are proactive, are knowledgeable about their health and their finances, and are willing to spend the time and energy to educate themselves and research their options.

If you are fortunate enough to have a company that provides more traditional comprehensive health insurance, you can consider enrolling in that plan. There may not be a deductible and services and medications are usually a fixed price, a co-pay, rather than a percentage of cost, or co-insurance. You don't need to worry as much about choosing to put off doctor visits, tests, and procedures, since deductibles aren't part of the plan.

Choose a high quality insurance plan accredited by the National Committee for Quality Assurance, NCQA. Not all insurance plans are created equal. Every year tens of thousands of people die prematurely simply because their plans didn't perform as well at keeping them as healthy as they could have.

Choose a high quality insurance plan accredited by the National Committee for Quality Assurance, NCQA.

In the end, understand the differences between deductible plans and traditional plans. Buy what you can afford. Understand that if you go without any coverage, you're relying on luck.

Office Visits

Your goal is to spend wisely and only to see the doctor when absolutely necessary. Don't confuse this with showing up to see your doctor only when you are practically dying! See your doctor when it's appropriate. To help you decide when medical care is appropriate, check www.familydoctor.org or purchase a health reference book. It may tell you how to care for the problem at home, and when to call the doctor.

> *The other important time to see your doctor is when routine testing is needed to screen for various cancers, high cholesterol, and diabetes.*

The other important time to see your doctor is when routine testing is needed to screen for various cancers, high cholesterol, and diabetes. Even healthy patients who have no symptoms and feel well should be checked out periodically. When and what test should be done depends on your age and gender. Refer to the previous section to figure out what tests you are due for. Problems found early, before you have symptoms, are more easily handled than when it's too late.

STAY HEALTHY

The ultimate goal is to stay healthy. After all, who enjoys seeing doctors, staying in hospitals, and feeling ill? To increase your chances of staying healthy, undergo screening tests and consider how your lifestyle and your choices impact your general well-being. Simple habits and choices are within your control: whether or not to smoke or drink alcoholic beverages, whether you stay active, protect yourself from unintentional injuries, and maintain a healthy weight. Most of us know the many risks associated with smoking and with drinking to excess. But do you know why staying active, protecting yourself from unintentional injuries, and maintaining a healthy weight are so important?

Stay Active

Research shows that improving health requires regular exercise. Strive to regularly engage in moderate-intensity physical activity for thirty minutes at least five times per week. At moderate intensity, a person feels that he is working "somewhat hard." This effort is similar to that of a healthy individual walking briskly, mowing the lawn, dancing, swimming, or biking on a level terrain.[188] At this level about 3.5 to 7 calories per minute are used. If you try a more vigorous activity, you can burn more than seven calories per minute. Regardless of your age, you can benefit from exercise.

If you are unable to begin with half an hour of moderate exercise, then build up do it. Start slowly. Depending on your overall health, a light walk for five or ten minutes might be all you are able to do. Make it easy enough so that you can do it. Make it a habit. Be proud of your accomplishment. As you get stronger, add more time to build up to thirty minutes. Don't get frustrated if you stop because you are too busy or forget. As they say, practice makes perfect, and it takes a lot of practice until regular physical activity becomes a habit.

Regular physical activity can improve cholesterol and decrease risk of developing high blood pressure, stroke, or diabetes. People who exercise also feel better about themselves and have fewer feelings of anxiety or depression. The majority of Americans don't get enough exercise to get health benefits.[189] Don't be one of them!

Protect Yourself

By maintaining a healthy weight, not smoking, monitoring and controlling your blood pressure, and undergoing the appropriate cancer screening tests, you will have decreased your risk of developing the first four leading causes of death for all ages (heart disease, cancer, stroke, and lower lung disease like

Unintentional injuries are the leading cause of death among people age one to thirty-four and the third leading cause among forty-five to fifty-four-year-olds. The most common cause of unintentional injuries is motor vehicle accidents.

emphysema).[190] The fifth leading cause of death is different. It has nothing to do with illness or infection but instead focuses on unintentional injuries.

Unintentional injuries are the leading cause of death among people age one to thirty-four and the third leading cause among forty-five to fifty-four-year-olds.[191] The most common cause of unintentional injuries is motor vehicle accidents. In 2002, the death rate for motor vehicle accidents was triple the HIV death rate and 60 percent of the breast cancer death rate.[192]

The number affected is significant. In the same year, among teenagers and young adults (fifteen to twenty-four years old), one-third of all deaths was due to motor vehicles accidents.[193] What is concerning is that among high school students, nearly one out of three rode with a driver who had been drinking. Being a passenger in a car with a potentially impaired driver was more common than not wearing seat belts (22 percent for high school males, 15 percent for females).

One study showed that the declining death rate in motor vehicle accidents over the past decade was not due to better drivers or improved roads, but to safer cars.

While seatbelt use dramatically decreases fatal injuries and moderate to critical injuries (45 and 50 percent, respectively), individuals can decrease their risk of dying from a motor vehicle accident by not riding with a driver who has had a drink, but also by thinking about what car they purchase and drive.

All vehicles are not created equal. Although they all seem strong with their metal frames, there are tangible engineering and design differences in motor vehicles. In an accident some protect their occupants better than others. The outcome could be life or death. The result could be walking away from an accident or a life filled with disability. Thinking critically about what you drive can impact your health. In fact, one study showed that the declining death rate in motor vehicle accidents over the past decade was not due to better drivers or improved roads, but to safer cars.[194]

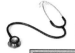 ## Real-Life Example

One month before my wedding, while driving to meet our pastor, our car spun out of control on the busiest Los Angeles freeway after hitting an oil spill. The car slammed into the hillside and flipped onto the driver's door. The vehicle was totaled and traffic was backed up for miles as emergency vehicles and personnel rushed to the scene.

Although my fiancée's father's car, his pride and joy, was a complete loss, it did during those critical seconds perform as it was designed. Detecting imminent impact, the seat belt tighteners activated, securing my fiancée and me. As parts of the car crumpled and absorbed the tremendous force of a sixty-mile-an-hour car stopping in a matter of a few yards, the steel cage held firm, protecting us from harm.

To this day I am convinced that had we been in another vehicle, one not optimally designed for safety, we could have been seriously injured or killed. Instead, my fiancée and I walked away, very much shaken, in shock, and grateful. Our wedding one month later was even more meaningful.

To learn more about car safety, check out the Insurance Institute for Highway Safety (IIHS) website at www.iihs.org and click on the vehicle ratings link to see how your car performs. An automaker's model safety rating often varies depending on the model year as well as whether optional features, like side airbags, were installed. IIHS is an independent nonprofit organization formed by the insurance industry and is dedicated to reducing death, injuries, and property damage from highway accidents.

Not all optional safety features save lives. Surprisingly, research has shown that antilock brakes have not decreased the number of crashes.[195] Perhaps it is because drivers, with the option, drive faster and brake later, thinking the technology enables them to do that. In fact, the feature minimizes the likelihood of skidding and losing control of the vehicle when driving on a slick surface. It does not necessarily shorten braking time or distance. If used prudently, it should in theory provide benefit.

Two safety options that have worked include using daytime running lights and electronic stability control (ESC) systems. The former has decreased the number of multiple vehicle daytime crashes and the latter has decreased fatal single vehicle accidents by 56 percent and all single vehicle crashes (nonfatal and fatal) by 40 percent.[196,197] ESC saves lives by preventing loss of control of the vehicle during emergency maneuvers or high speed turns on slippery surfaces. It works by having a computer, equipped with sensors, assist with braking individual wheels, instead of having all wheels lock-up, in order to gain maximum traction and control for the driver to keep the car on the road. It is expected that by 2012 all new vehicles will be equipped with electronic stability control systems as it is estimated to save 10,000 lives annually out of the 34,000 fatal crashes and prevent up to 252,000 injuries every year.[198,199] For this feature, the added cost is $111 per vehicle if it already has antilock brakes.[200]

Drive sober, wear your seat belt, and sit in a vehicle equipped with safety features designed to maximize survival and minimize injury. Also remember not to speed and to drive safely.

Maintain a Healthy Weight

About two-thirds of Americans are considered overweight or obese. Sadly, even our children are becoming heavier and developing illnesses like diabetes at younger ages. Should this trend continue, the next generation of Americans will be the first to not live as long as their parents. Being too heavy cuts your life short.

To figure out if you are overweight or obese, calculate your body mass index or BMI by going to www.cdc.gov and searching for BMI. You need to know your height and weight. As indicated in a previous section, the formula is as follows:

weight (in pounds)/height ^{2} (in inches) times 703

or

weight (in kilograms)/height ^{2} (in meters)

Overweight is defined as a BMI of 25 to 29.9 and obesity is a BMI of 30 or greater. A normal BMI is 18.5 to 24.9. A BMI of less than 18.5 is considered underweight.

While a BMI by itself doesn't mean that an individual is unhealthy, it does correlate with body fat. It is not completely accurate; athletes may have a higher BMI since muscle weighs more than fat, and older patients and women have more fat at any given BMI. Nevertheless, calculating a BMI is quick and easy for you and can help you and your doctor begin the discussion about your health. Your BMI is a number you can control directly with weight loss.

Americans are overweight or obese because of our hectic and sedentary lifestyles. We spend more and more time in our cars, watching television, or using the Internet and playing computer games than we do exercising or cooking for ourselves after a long

About two-thirds of Americans are considered overweight or obese. Should this trend continue, the next generation of Americans will be the first to not live as long as their parents.

day. Instead we opt to go out and get food. Unfortunately, as we have become less active, the serving sizes of the foods we eat have increased dramatically. Check out an eye-opening and fun quiz that not only shows how portion sizes have ballooned over the past twenty years, but also how much exercise we need to burn off that excess in calories. The Portion Distortion quiz by the National Heart Lung and Blood Institute is at http://hp2010.nhlbihin.net/portion.

The first question notes that twenty years ago a bagel was three inches wide and had 140 calories. Today a bagel is six inches wide and contains a heftier 350 calories. To burn off those extra calories, a person weighing 130 pounds would need to rake leaves for fifty minutes.[201] To lose weight, he would have to do even more exercise. The test will help you rethink how to approach eating and the need to control portion sizes. If you don't take control of how you eat, no one else will.

If you need to lose weight, check out the Obesity Education Initiative and look for the "Aim for a Healthy Weight" link at www.nhlbi.nih. gov/about/oei. There are plenty of tips for shopping for healthy food, getting more physical activity, making behavioral changes, and other helpful advice.

If you are overweight or obese, even a small amount of weight loss is beneficial. Cutting down on your food portions is an easy way to start. One way to do this is to use a smaller dinner plate. Another is to take an empty regular sized frozen dinner entrée tray and use it to determine how much food to eat. Check with your doctor if you are concerned about how to lose weight or wondering if your plan will affect your health. Congratulations for taking that important first step.

USING THE INTERNET FOR RESEARCH

When I started medical school, the Internet was still in its infancy. We hardly encountered patients with printouts about their medical problems, lists of medication side effects, or alternative therapies.

Those days are over. Today, patients have a wealth of medical knowledge easily accessible at the touch of a few keystrokes. Doctors, too, can use the technology to look up references and review the latest medical guidelines and research without needing to search through piles of journals or textbooks. Much as the Internet is being used to change the way we all communicate, shop, and plan, it will also transform the way patients and physicians interact and how health care is delivered.

An excellent free reference, the Merck Manual of Medical Information Home Edition, can be found at www.merck. com/mmhe.

However, as with all new technology, there are some tradeoffs. The Internet is not regulated. Anyone can put up a website touting a medical therapy which may sound good but is not scientifically proven. Others point out known, uncommon complications and side effects of medical procedures and prescription medications, exaggerating the consequences and potentially scaring the general public.

I am all for educating the public and empowering the public with more information. However, if you use the Internet to do your research, begin with the websites found in this book. I have personally reviewed each of them to ensure that they are factually correct. Also refer to websites run by reputable organizations including your local medical school and other medical groups.

An excellent free reference, started in 1997, the *Merck Manual of Medical Information Home Edition,* can be found at www.merck.com/ mmhe. It provides easy-to-understand language and enough information to help anyone researching an illness. Since 1899, Merck, the pharmaceutical company, has been producing a medical text called the *Merck Manual of Diagnosis and Therapy,* which is used by many medical students and physicians (including yours truly).

Another good place to start is at www.medlineplus.gov, which features information on hundreds of health topics, a drug and supplement database, a medical dictionary and encyclopedia, interactive tutorials, videos on many surgical procedures, and a link to clinical trials. The National Library of Medicine, which is a part of the National Institutes of Health, is the agency providing the information.

If you need to find out more about cancer, three websites that are helpful include the National Cancer Institute at www.cancer.gov, the American Cancer Society at www.cancer.org, and People Living with Cancer at www.plwc.org, which is sponsored by the American Society of Clinical Oncologists.

While you should not completely disregard other websites, take their information and see if you can corroborate it with information from trusted sources. Finally, if you aren't sure, ask your doctor. Better yet, email him!

THE FUTURE OF AMERICA'S HEALTH CARE

In an ideal world, all Americans would have health care. We would choose our medical care based on our personal preference rather than on our ability to pay. We would never worry about going bankrupt to help a loved one get medical care.

In an ideal world, an individual's medical information, including past medical history, medications, allergies, and office visits would be stored on a secure computer database easily accessible by physicians either down the street or across the country. Physicians and patients would be supported by systems that promoted good health, delivered the latest and most effective treatments, and reminded all of us, despite our busy schedules, to remember to get preventive screening tests. Treatments would be based not on marketing, but on proven therapies. Future medications would be tailor-made for our specific ailments and genetic makeup. Americans could claim to live the longest and have the highest quality of life in the world.

Sadly, this is not the state of the American healthcare system. Will this ideal world ever occur in our lifetime?

I don't know. I do know that our current healthcare system favors those who are prudent and prepared. But regardless of what our future healthcare system looks like, I hope the knowledge you've gained will keep you healthy and well today and in the future.

TAKE-HOME POINTS

✓ *Absolutely vital to staying healthy financially is to have health insurance* to protect from, at the very minimum, catastrophic financial hardship incurred by a major illness or accident. To improve your health, if you have an option, choose an insurance plan that is highly rated by NCQA.

✓ *Going to the doctor's office when it is necessary, even at times when you feel perfectly well,* is important to staying healthy. To help you decide when medical care is needed, check out www.familydoctor.org.

✓ *You have the greatest responsibility to keeping yourself healthy.* This includes staying active, protecting yourself from car accidents and other unintentional injuries, and maintaining a healthy weight.

✓ *Unintentional injuries are the leading cause of death among people ages one to thirty-four and the third leading cause among forty-five to fifty-four-year-olds.* The most common cause is motor vehicle accidents. Consider purchasing a car based on its safety rating. The likelihood of having a lifetime of disability versus walking away from an accident relies on differences in engineering and safety design of the vehicle.

✓ *The American healthcare system is in crisis.* Our current system favors those with the knowledge about how to stay healthy and who know how to select the right care. Hopefully, after reading this book, you are now one of these wise patients.

Referenced Websites

THE DOCTOR IS IN

PART ONE: The Most Important Policy You Will Ever Own

Do I Qualify for an HSA?

www.irs.gov

The Quality of Your Health Insurance Plan Quality Matters!

www.ncqa.org

www.usnews.com/healthplans

www.consumerreports.org

www.leapfroggroup.org

You're on Your Own

www.dol.gov/ebsa/faqs

www.ehealthinsurance.com

www.nationalhealthstore.com

PART TWO: Mastering the Ten-Minute Doctor Office Visit

Don't See Your Doctor

www.familydoctor.org

PART THREE: Do the Right Thing Regularly and Repeatedly

American Cancer Society (ACS)

www.cancer.org

Breast Cancer Screening

www.komen.org/bse

www.fda.gov/cdrh

www.cancer.gov/bcrisktool

Testicular Cancer

www.fda.gov/fdac, search for testicular self-exam

American Heart Association (AHA)

www.americanheart.org

High Cholesterol

www.nhlbi.nih.gov/guidelines/cholesterol

American Diabetes Association (ADA)

www.cdc.gov, search for BMI

www.diabetes.org

U. S. Preventive Services Task Force (USPSTF)

www.ahrq.gov,

find the U.S. Preventive Services Task Force link (USPSTF)

Immunizations and Vaccinations

www.cdc.gov/vaccines/programs/vfc

www.cdc.gov/vaccines

| PART FOUR: | Meet Your Medical Team |

Importance of Board Certification

www.abms.org

Licensing

www.fsmb.org

Internists and Family Physicians

www.abim.org
www.theabfm.org

Specialists

www.abms.org
www.abim.org

Medical Specialties

Allergist/Immunologist — www.aaaai.org, www.acaai.org

Cardiologist — www.acc.org

Dermatologist — www.aad.org

Endocrinologist — www.endo-society.org

Gastroenterologist — www.acg.gi.org

Hematologist/Oncologist — www.hematology.org

Nephrologist — www.asn-online.org

Neurologist — www.aan.com

Pulmonologist — www.chestnet.org

Rheumatologist — www.rheumatology.org

Surgical Specialties

General Surgeon — www.facs.org

Ophthalmologist — www.aao.org

Orthopedist — www.aaos.org

Otolaryngologist — www.aboto.org

Other Primary Care Fields

Obstetrician/Gynecologist — www.acog.org

Pediatrician — www.aap.org

Emergency Medicine

Emergency Medicine Physicians — www.acep.org

Psychiatry

Psychiatrist — www.healthyminds.org, www.psych.org

What's the Deal with DOs (Doctor of Osteopathic Medicine)?

Other Providers

Physician Assistants (PAs) — www.aapa.org

Nurse Practitioners (NPs) — www.aanp.org

PART FIVE: The Truth About Medications

Generic and Branded Medications: What's the Difference?

www.crbestbuydrugs.org

www.fda.gov/cder/ogd

Making Sense of Over-the-Counter (OTC) Medications

www.fda.gov/cder/audiences

www.medlineplus.gov

Other Resources for Paying for Prescription Medications

www.togetherrxaccess.com

PART SIX: | Caveat Emptor, Or "Let the Buyer Beware"

Herbal and Dietary Supplements

www.naturalstandard.com

www.consumerreportsmedicalguide.org

PART SEVEN: | Twenty-First Century Medical Care

PART EIGHT: | Take Control: Excellent Health Pays

Office Visits

www.familydoctor.org

Protect Yourself

www.iihs.org

Maintain a Healthy Weight

www.cdc.gov, search for BMI

http://hp2010.nhlbihin.net/portion

www.nhlbi.nih.gov/about/oei, look for the Aim for a Healthy
Weight link

Using the Internet for Research

www.merck.com/mmhe

www.medlineplus.gov

www.cancer.gov

www.cancer.org

www.plwc.org

NOTES

Introduction

1. The Kaiser Family Foundation and Health Educational Trust, "Employer Health Benefits 2005 Summary of Findings," Document 7316: 1.

2. "Public Opinion: The Public on Health Care Costs," *Kaiser Health Poll Report*: December 2005: 1.

3. National Committee for Quality Assurance, "The State of Health Care Quality," 2005.

4. Employee Benefits Research Institute Press Release, "Average Couple Today Needs $295,000 for Retiree Health Expenses," PR# 742, July 20, 2006.

5. H Gleckman, "Your New Health Plan," *Businessweek*, 8 November 2004, p. 88–98.

6. The Kaiser Family Foundation and Health Educational Trust, "Employer Health Benefits 2006 Annual Survey," Publication 7527: 106.

7. Employee Benefit Research Institute—The Commonwealth Fund, "Consumer-Driven Health Plans Slow to Catch On, 2nd Annual Survey Finds New Plans Also Not a Major Source of Coverage for the Uninsured," Press Release December 7, 2006, # 755: 2.

8. "The First National Report Card on Quality of Health Care in America," RAND Health, RB-9053, 2004, http://www.rand.org/publications/RB/RB9053/RB9053.pdf

9. National Coalition on Health Care, "Facts on Health Insurance Quality," www.nchc. org (accessed 10/4/2003).

PART ONE: The Most Important Policy You Will Ever Own

10. Employee Benefit Research Institute Notes, "2006 Health Confidence Survey: Dissatisfaction with Healthcare System Doubles Since 1998," November 2006, Vol. 27, No. 11.

11. Except in Massachusetts where in April 2006 a law was enacted requiring all residents to have health insurance. Many other states since then have proposed various plans with some mandating all residents enroll in a health insurance plan.

12. NBC's *Dateline*, "Critical Condition," originally aired August 6, 2004.

13. Employee Benefit Research Institute Notes, "2005 Health Confidence Survey: Cost and Quality Not Linked," November 2005, Vol. 26, No. 11.

14. See note 6 above.

15. "Public Perceptions of Costs for Health Care Products and Services Differ Widely," *The Wall Street Journal Online/Harris Interactive Health Care Poll*, July 19, 2004, Vol. 3, Issue 13.

16. Employee Benefit Research Institute Notes, "Survey of Consumer-Driven Health Plans Raises Issues," February 2006, Vol. 27, No. 2.

17. Kaiser Family Foundation, "National Survey of Enrollees in Consumer Directed Health Plans," November 2006, Publication #7594.

18. See note 16 above.

19. See note 17 above.

20. Highlights of 2003 Tax Changes, Department of the Treasury Internal Revenue Service, Publication 553 (rev. January 2004), Catalog 15101G: 7-10.

21. "HMO or PPO Picking a Managed-Care Plan," *Consumer Reports*, October 2003: 35-39.

22. Publication 969, *Health Savings Accounts and Other Tax-Favored Health Plans*, Department of the Treasury Internal Revenue Service, 2005.

23. IRS Publication 502, Cat. 15002Q, *Medical and Dental Expenses*, 2.

24. Melynda Wilcox, "When Insurance Makes You Sick," *Kiplinger's*, September 2003: 74-77.

25. "The First National Report Card on Quality of Health Care in America," RAND Health, RB-9053, 2004, http://www.rand.org/publications/RB/RB9053/RB9053.pdf

26. S. Smith, "Care for Heart-Attack Patients Vary, Federal Study Finds," *Boston Globe*, June 24, 2003.

27. "Medical Care Often Not Optimal, Study Finds," *Washington Post*, June 26, 2003, Nation section, A02.

28. For comparison, note that the American Cancer Society estimated that in 2005, over 40,000 women would die of breast cancer, the second leading cause of cancer deaths among women.

29. "HMOs Bringing Back Restrictions, Survey Finds," Reuters, http://www.msnbc.msn.com/id/5670810, August 11, 2004.

30. http://story.news.yahoo.com/news?tmpl=story&u=/nm/20040902/hl_nm/health_hospital_quality_dc

31. C. Pesman, "Three Sure Cures for Medical Sticker Shock," *Money*, April 2006: 46.

32. E. Kountze, "Steppingstone Jobs for Recent Grads," *Kiplinger's Personal Finance*, August 2004: 107-108.

33. L. Rapaport, "Region Feels Pain of High Hospital Bills," *Sacramento Bee*, November 10, 2002.

34. "Uninsured Patients Pay More for Care," Associated Press, June 24, 2004, http://www.msnbc.com/id/5290172/print/1/displaymode/1098/ (accessed August 8, 2004).

35. R. Helman, et al., "Public Attitudes on the U.S. Healthcare System: Findings from the Health Confidence Survey," *Employee Benefit Research Institute*, November 2004, Issue Brief No. 275.

36. http://www.healthpartners.com/empower/costofcare (accessed October 27, 2004).

37. http://www.cms.hhs.gov/healthcareconinit/ (accessed June 23, 2006).

38. "Medicaid: A Brief Summary," http://www.cms.hhs.gov/publications/overview-medicare-medicaid/default4.asp (accessed August 8, 2004).

39. http://www.nchc.org/facts/coverage.shtml (accessed February 15, 2007), referring to the age group of adults between 25 to 64 years of age.

PART TWO: Mastering the Ten-Minute Office Doctor Office Visit

40.   "The Effect of Physician Behavior on the Collection of Data," *Annals of Internal Medicine 101*, no. 5 November 1984: 692-96.

41.   "Are Patients' Office Visits with Physicians Getting Shorter?" *NEJM*, Vol. 344, No.3, January 18, 2001: 198-204.

42.   National Ambulatory Medical Care Survey, 2001, Centers of Disease Control and Prevention.

43.   Harrison's Principles of Internal Medicine Companion Handbook, 14th edition, Fauci et al., McGraw-Hill, 1998: 554.

44.   Kiplinger's Personal Finance, September 2003: 26.

45.   *Modern Medicine*, March 1997, Vol. 65, issue 3.

PART THREE: Do the Right Thing Regularly and Repeatedly

46.   http://www.bartleby.com/100/245.html (accessed March 29, 2006).

47.   S. Oboler, et al., "Public Expectations and Attitudes for Annual Physical Examinations and Testing," *Annals of Internal Medicine*, Vol. 136, No. 9, May 7, 2002: 652-659.

48.   "Tests to Find Cancer Early," Chart (accessed March 20, 2006), at http://www.cancer.org/docroot/PRO/PRO_4_2_ColonMD_Educating_Patients.asp

49.   Ibid.

50.   Ibid

51.   R. Rubin, "Injected into Controversy," *USA Today*, October 20, 2005, Life section: 8d.

52.   K. Gaither, et al., "An Evaluation of Perceived Patient Misconception—Was a Pap Smear Performed?" Acad Emerg Med 2001, 8: 543.

53.   Cancer Statistics 2005, American Cancer Society.

54.   R. Rubin, "Study finds mammograms not as frequent as thought," *USA Today*, September 12, 2005, Life section: 7.

55.   See note 48 above.

56.   "Screening for Breast Cancer," *AHRQ Publication No. APPIP02-0016*, February 2002.

57.   "Digital Mammography Trial Results Announced: Women with Dense Breasts, Women Younger than 50, and Those Who are Perimenopausal May Benefit from Digital Mammograms," http://www.cancer.gov/newscenter/pressreleases/DMISTrelease (accessed 4/3/2006).

58.   See note 53 above.

59.   See note 48 above.

60.   Ibid.

61.   National Cancer Institute Fact Sheet, "The Prostate-Specific Antigen (PSA) Test: Questions and Answers," reviewed 8/17, 2004, http://www.cancer.gov/cancertopics/factsheet/Detection/PSA (accessed 4/3/2006).

62. "Inventor of PSA Cancer Test Says It's Overused," http://story.news.yahoo.com/news?tmpl=story&u=/nm/20040910/hl_nm/cancer_test_dc

63. http://www.cancer.org/docroot/CRI/content/CRI_2_4_3X_Can_prostate_cancer_be_found_early_36.asp?rnav=cri (accessed 4/3/2006).

64. J.M. Walsh, et al., "Colon cancer screening in the ambulatory setting," *Preventive Medicine*, 35: 209-218, 2002.

65. American Cancer Society's Cancer Facts and Figures 2002.

66. See note 53 above.

67. http://www.cancer.org/docroot/CRI/content/CRI_2_4_2X_What_are_the_risk_factors_for_colon_and_rectum_cancer.asp?sitearea= (accessed December 23, 2005).

68. See note 53 above.

69. http://www.americanheart.org/presenter.jhtml?identifier=2139 (accessed December 23, 2005).

70. http://www.nhlbi.nih.gov/about/framingham/index.html accessed (April 3, 2006).

71. *Diabetes Care*, Vol 29, Supplement 1, January 2006.

72. Ibid.

73. http://www.cdc.gov/nccdphp/dnpa/obesity/index.htm (accessed May 22, 2006).

74. http://www.ahcpr.gov/clinic/uspstfab.htm (accessed November, 19, 2005).

75. *The Guide to Clinical Preventive Services 2005, Recommendations of the U.S. Preventive Services Task Force.*

76. http://www.cdc.gov/nip/diseases/measles/faqs.htm (accessed May 13, 2006).

77. http://www.cdc.gov/nip/diseases/measles/history.htm#HOM (accessed May 13, 2006).

78. http://www.bt.cdc.gov/agent/smallpox/training/overview/, from Module 1, History and Epidemiology of Global Smallpox Eradication (accessed November 25, 2005).

79. A. Manning, "Not all children are getting recommended pneumococcal vaccine, *USA Today*, September 2, 2003, Life section: 7d.

80. http://www.cdc.gov/nip/publications/pink/tetanus.pdf (accessed December 24, 2005).

81. A. Manning, "Doctors hope new shots will get parents to bring older children in," *USA Today*, March 8, 2005, Life section: 7d.

82. Ibid.

83. HPV Vaccination Information Statement (interim), 9/5/06 (accessed December 28, 2006), from www.cdc.gov/nip.

84. http://www.cdc.gov/nip/publications/VIS/vis-PneumoConjugate.pdf, (accessed July 8, 2006).

85. http://www.cdc.gov/ncidod/dbmd/diseaseinfo/streppneum_t.htm (accessed July 8, 2006).

86. http://www.cdc.gov/flu/keyfacts.htm (accessed July 8, 2006).

87. "Prevention and Control of Influenza: Recommendations of the Advisory Committee on Immunization Practices (ACIP)," *MMWR, Morbidity and Mortality Weekly Report*, CDC, (July 28, 2006), Vol. 55, RR-10.

PART FOUR: Meet Your Medical Team

88.   *A System in Need of Change: Restructuring Federal Health Care Policy to Make Patient-Centered Care Available to All, State of the Nation's Health Care: 2007,* The American College of Physicians, January 22, 2007.

89.   "The Impending Collapse of Primary Care Medicine and Its Implications for the State of the Nation's Health Care," *A Report from the American College of Physicians,* January 30, 2006.

90.   Ibid.

91.   Ibid.

92.   Ibid.

93.   Ibid.

94.   Greenwald and Associates, "2005 Health Confidence Survey," Employee Benefits Research Institute, Notes, November 2005, No. 26, Vol. 11.

95.   http://www.abim.org/resources/statcert.shtm#2 (accessed February 19, 2005).

96.   http://www.ama-assn.org/vapp/freida/srch/1,1239,,00.html (accessed June 12, 2005).

97.   www.osteopathic.org (accessed June 11, 2005).

98.   www.aapa.org (accessed April 24, 2005).

99.   www.aanp.org, (accessed April 24, 2005).

100.   D. Stires, "Technology Has Transformed the VA," *Fortune,* May 15, 2006 (accessed September 18, 2006), http://money.cnn.com/magazines/fortune/fortune_archive/2006/05/15/8376846/index.htm

101.   S. Lohr, "Is Kaiser the Future of American Health Care?" *New York Times,* October 31, 2004, at http://www.nytimes.com/2004/10/31/business/yourmoney/31hmo.html?pagewanted=3&ei=5090&en=c2e37a34cde40ed8&ex=1256875200&partner=rssuserl and, (accessed on April 15, 2007).

PART FIVE: The Truth About Medications

102.   http://www.pdabell.com/quotes/quotes_list_sub.php?subject=Medicine (accessed January 14, 2006).

103.   http://www.britannica.com/ebc/article-9374205?query=william%20osler&ct= (accessed January 14, 2006).

104.   A. Gardner, "Cost-Cutting on Drugs Has Health Cost," www.healthcentral.com (accessed October 16, 2004).

105.   "Prescription Drug Expenditures in 2001: Another Year of Escalating Costs," The National Institute for Health Care Management Research and Educational Foundation, May 2002.

106.   Ibid.

107.   "Prescription Drugs and Mass Media Advertising, 2000," The National Institute for Health Care Management Research and Educational Foundation, November 2001.

108.   Ibid.

109. Ibid.

110. F. Sierles, et al., "Medical Students' Exposure to and Attitudes About Drug Company Interactions: A National Survey," *JAMA*, 9/7/2005, Vol. 294 Issue 9:1034-1042.

111. A. Pollack, "Stanford to Ban Drug Makers' Gifts to Doctors, Even Pens," http://www. nytimes.com/2006/09/12/business/12drug.html?ei=5070&en=e5411fe29a70b439 &ex=1159675200&adxnnl=1&adxnnlx=1159556712-g6xrt1+bqE2nHp+2rzVUkw (accessed September 29, 2006).

112. Center for Drug Evaluation and Research, Generic Drugs: Questions and Answers, http://www.fda.gov/cder/consumerinfo/generics_q&a.htm#whatare, (accessed May 19, 2006).

113. http://www.fda.gov/cder/consumerinfo/generic_text.htm (accessed January 14,2006).

114. "Generic Anti-Seizure Med May Not Be as Effective," http://news.yahoo.com (accessed October 28, 2004), referring to Neurology, October 26, 2004.

115. B. Mintzes, et al., "Influence of direct to consumer pharmaceutical advertising in patients' requests on prescribing decisions: two sites cross sectional survey," *BMJ*, February 2, 2002, 324: 278-279.

116. www.excedrin.com (accessed January 9, 2006).

117. http://www.pfizerch.com/product.aspx?id=459 (accessed October 11, 2006).

118. http://www.pfizerch.com/brand.aspx?id=34 (accessed May 13, 2006).

119. www.robitussin.com (accessed May 13, 2006).

120. www.sudafed.com (accessed May 13, 2006).

121. www.tylenol.com (accessed January 9, 2006).

PART SIX: Caveat Emptor, Or "Let the Buyer Beware"

122. "Attorney General Demands That Coca-Cola, Nestle Prove Claims Of 'Calorie-Burning' Beverage,"

Connecticut Attorney General's Office Press Release, February 5, 2007, http://www. ct.gov/ag/cwp/view.asp?A=2788&Q=331994 (accessed March 9, 2007).

123. Julie Silver, MD, "One Doctor's Journey into Concierge Medicine, Unique Opportunities," *The Physician's Resource*, Sep/Oct 2003.

124. Carol Smith, "In retainer medicine, the doctor is always in," *Seattle Post-Intelligencer*, Thursday, July 5, 2001.

125. Liz Kowalczyk, "Boutique Care Is Coming for Wealthy Patients at Boston-Area Hospital," *The Boston Globe*, August 11, 2003.

126. Susan Meyers, "Concierge Medicine—Who Really Pays for Gold Standard Access to Doctors," *Trustee*, January 2003: 13-19.

127. William Hoffman, "Fed up, some doctors turn to boutique medicine," *ACP-ASIM Observer*, October 2001.

128. T.A. Brennan, "Luxury Primary Care—Market Innovation or Threat to Access?" *New England Journal of Medicine*, Volume 346:1165-1168, 15: April 11, 2002.

129. See note 125 above.

130. See note 127 above.

131. Nancy Luna "The doctor is in … for a price," *Orange County Register*, January 11, 2004.

132. "Concierge physicians form national trade organization," *Modern Healthcare*, Vol. 34, Issue 9, page 46, March 1, 2004.

133. Michael Romano, "Concierge critique," *Modern Healthcare*, Vol. 34, Issue 15, p8, 1c, April 12, 2004.

134. John D. Goodson, MD, "New Practice designs deviate from tradition," Ethics Forum, November 3, 2003, www.ama.assn.org/amednews/2003/11/03/prcc1103.htm

135. C. Dennis O'Hare, MD, Msc, and John Corlett, "The Outcomes of Open-Access Scheduling," *Family Practice Management*, February 2004, Vol. 11, No.2, 35-38.

136. Dorothy L. Pennachio, "Full-body scans – or scams?" *Medical Economics*, August 2002.

137. Whole Body Scanning Using Computed Tomography, FDA website, www.fda.gov/dfrh/ct/

138. HealthView website, http://www.healthview.com/about.htm

139. See note 136 above.

140. Ibid.

141. See note 137 above.

142. Dr. David Kessler, "Commentary: Use of full-body scans by healthy people," "Morning Edition," NPR, June 4, 2002.

143. Judy Peres, "Cancer Study Is Skeptical about Value of High-Tech Body Scans," *Chicago Tribune*, January 15, 2003.

144. www.cnn.com/2003/HEALTH/12/01/virtual.colonoscopu.ap/index.html

145. www.pbs.org/newshour/bb/health/july-dec03/colonoscopy_12-02.html

146. "Virtual colonoscopy needs to improve before widespread clinical use," *Cancer Weekly*, April 27, 2004, 82-83.

147. M. Zoler, "Opinions Still Divided on Role of Coronary Calcium," *Family Practice News*, October 1, 2003, 29.

148. G. Kolata, "New Studies Question Value of Opening Arteries," *New York Times*, Health, March 21, 2004.

149. W. Boden, et al., "Optimal Medical Therapy with or without PCI for Stable Coronary Disease," *New England Journal of Medicine*, Number 15,Volume 356:1503-1516, April 12, 2007.

150. See note 148 above.

151. L. Szabo, "Study Stirs Debate Over Full-body Scan's Cancer Risk," *USA Today*, August 31, 2004, 1A.

152. www.fda.gov, Acting FDA Commissioner Dr. Lester M. Crawford Outlines Science-Based Plan for Dietary Supplement Enforcement – April 19, 2004.

153. www.about.com, Annual U.S. Video Game Sales: The NPD Group Reports on Video Game Sales and Best Selling Video Game Titles.

154. www.premierecapital.nct, Digitalcinema partners.

155. Correspondence – Herbal Medicine, *NEJM*, 348: 15, April 10, 2003, 1498-1500.

156. Overview of Dietary Supplements, U.S. Food and Drug Administration, Center for Food Safety and Applied Nutrition, January 3, 2001, www.cfsan.fda.gov~/dms/ds-oview.html.

157. http://www.cfsan.fda.gov/~dms/supplmnt.html (accessed March 12, 2006).

158. Peter A.G. M. De Smet, "Herbal Remedies," *NEJM*, Vol. 347, No. 25, December 19, 2002, 2046-2056.

159. "Too Risky: Government Announces Ban on Herbal Supplement Ephedra," http://sportsillustrated.cnn.com/2003/baseball/mlb/12/30/ephedra.ban.ap

160. FDA Issues Regulation Prohibiting Sale of Dietary Supplements Containing Ephedrine Alkaloids and Reiterates Its Advice That Consumers Stop Using These Products, www.fda.gov/bbs/topics/NEWS/2003/NEW01021.html

161. FDA Announces Rule Prohibiting Sale of Dietary Supplements Containing Ephedrine Alkaloids Effective April 12, www.fda.gov/bbs/topics/NEWS/2004/NEW01050.html.

162. U.S. Warns About Impotence Product Sold on Web http://story.news.yahoo.com/news?tmpl=story&u=/nm/20041102/hl_nm/health_impotence_dc (accessed November 2, 2004).

163. M. Planta, "Increased Education Is Needed About Use of Herbal Products," *American Family Physician,* December 1999, Vol. 60, No. 9, 2630.

164. "Dangerous Supplements Still at Large," *Consumer Reports*, May 2004, 12-17.

165. T. Kirn, "Group Rates Efficacy of Herbs," *Family Practice News,* April 15, 2004, Vol. 34, No. 8, 1, 26.

166. C. Adams, "More Research Is Questioning Safety, Effectiveness of Herbs," *Wall Street Journal*, August 29, 2002.

167. A. Shaughnessy, "Glucosamine and Chondroitin for Osteoarthritis," *American Family Physician*, December 1, 2003, 2244.

168. D. O. Clegg, et al., "Glucosamine, Chondroitin Sulfate, and the Two in Combination for Painful Knee Osteoarthritis," *New England Journal of Medicine,* February 23, 2006, Vol. 354: 795 -808.

169. "Antioxidants and Disease Prevention: Should We All Take Supplements?" *Consultant*, August 2003, 1084. Vitamin E May Do More Harm Than Good, Study Finds.

170. http://story.news.yahoo.com/news?tmpl=story&u=/nm/20041110/hl_nm/health_heart_vitamin_dc

171. http://story.news.yahoo.com/news?tmpl=story&u=/acs/20050315/hl_acs/study__vitamin_e_no_help_against_cancer

172. See note 166 above.

PART SEVEN: Twenty-First Century Medical Care

173. RM, Wachter, and L. Goldman, "The Emerging Role of "Hospitalists" in the American Healthcare system," *New England Journal of Medicine*, Volume 335:514-517, Number 7: August 15, 1996.

174. S. Frost, F. Michota, "Hospital Medicine: Past, Present, and Future," *Primary Care Reports*, August 2003, Vol. 9, Number 8, 75-84.

175. RM Wachter, "Hospitalists in the United States – Mission Accomplished or Work in Progress?" *New England Journal of Medicine*, Volume 350:1935-1936, Number 19: May 6, 2004.

176. E. Noffsinger, and J. Scott, "Understanding Today's Group Visit Models," *Group Practice Journal*, Group Practice Journal, February 2000, 46-58.

177. Ibid.

178. Ibid.

179. Ibid.

180. Ibid

181. Ibid.

182. S. Houck, et al., "Group Visits 101," *Family Practice Management*, May 2003, 66-68.

183. S. Masley, et al., "Planning Group Visits for High-Risk Patients," *Family Practice Management*, June 2000.

184. B. White, "Making Evidence-based Medicine Doable in Everyday Practice," *Family Practice Management*, February 2004, 51-58.

185. J. Manson and K. Martin, "Postmenopausal Hormone-Replacement Therapy," *NEJM*, Vol. 345: 1, July 5, 2001, 34-40.

186. H. Nelson, et al., "Postmenopausal Hormone Replacement Therapy – Scientific Review," *JAMA*, Vol. 288, No. 7, August 21, 2002, 872-881.

PART EIGHT: Take Control: Excellent Health Pays

187. A. Kadet, et al., "Double Your Money," *SmartMoney*, March 2007, p 69.

188. http://www.cdc.gov/nccdphp/dnpa/physical/terms/index.htm#Moderate (accessed April 25, 2006).

189. http://www.cdc.gov/nccdphp/dnpa/physical/importance/index.htm (accessed July 3, 2006).

190. Chartbook on Trends in the Health of Americans, Health, United States, 2005, Hyattsville, Maryland: 2005, 68.

191. National Center for Injury Prevention and Control, http://webappa.cdc.gov/sasweb/ncipc/leadcaus10.html (accessed January 30, 2006).

192. Table 29, Age-adjusted death rates for select causes of death, according to sex, race, and Hispanic origin: United States, selected years 1950-2002, National Center for Health Statistics, Health, United States, 2005, With Chart book on Trends in the Health of Americans, Hyattsville, Maryland: 2005, 170.

193. National Center for Health Statistics, Health, United States, 2005, With Chart book on Trends in the Health of Americans, Hyattsville, Maryland: 2005, 36.

194. "Declining Death Rates due to Safer Vehicles, Not Better Drivers or Improving Roadways," News Release, August 10, 2006 (accessed on October 20, 2006) www.iihs.org

195. http://www.iihs.org/research/qanda/antilock.html (accessed January 30, 2006).

196. http://www.iihs.org/research/qanda/drl.html (accessed January 30, 2006).

197. Status Report Newsletter Vol. 40., No. 1, January 3, 2005, available at www.iihs.org.

198. "DOT Proposes Anti-Rollover Technology for New Vehicles," National Highway Traffic and Safety Administration, press release, September 14, 2006, (accessed at www.nhtsa.gov October 20, 2006).

199. "Electronic Stability Control Could Prevent Nearly One Third of All Fatal Crashes and Reduce Rollover Risk by as Much as 80%," News Release, June 13, 2006, www.iihs.org (accessed October 20, 2006).

200. "U.S. Department of Transportation Secretary Mary E. Peters Announces A Substantial Life-Saving Technology for All New Passenger Vehicles," Press Release April 5, 2007, www.dot.gov/affairs/dot3707.htm (accessed April 19, 2007).

201. http://hp2010.nhlbihin.net/portion/ (accessed July 3, 2006).

INDEX

X